AN INTEGRATIVE METAREGRESSION
FRAMEWORK FOR DESCRIPTIVE
EPIDEMIOLOGY

Publications on Global Health

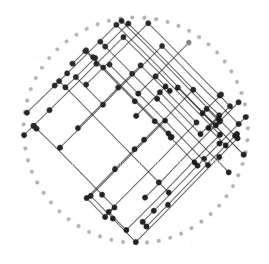

AN INTEGRATIVE METAREGRESSION

FRAMEWORK FOR DESCRIPTIVE

EPIDEMIOLOGY

EDITED BY ABRAHAM D. FLAXMAN,

THEO VOS, AND CHRISTOPHER J.L. MURRAY

UNIVERSITY OF WASHINGTON PRESS

Seattle and London

University of Washington Press

www.washington.edu/uwpress

Library of Congress Cataloging-in-Publication Data

An integrative metaregression framework for descriptive epidemiology / edited by Abraham D. Flaxman, Theo Vos, and Christopher J.L. Murray.

    p.   cm.

  Includes bibliographical references and index.

  ISBN 978-0-295-99184-9 (hardcover : alk. paper)

  I. Flaxman, Abraham D., editor.   II. Vos, Theo, Dr., editor. III. Murray, Christopher J.L., editor.

  [DNLM: 1. Global Burden of Diseases, Injuries, and Risk Factors Study 2010. 2. Epidemiology. 3. Global Health—statistics & numerical data. 4. Models, Statistical. 5. Meta-Analysis as Topic. WA 900.1]

  RA652

  614.4—dc23

2015016435

Contents

Figures

Contents

Tables

Acknowledgments

The material in this book could not have been developed without the vast and sustained support of a large number of people. Many have been so important to the project that it is a great pleasure to thank them specifically here. Project officer Rebecca Cooley was essential to shepherding this project in its earliest days, and post-graduate fellows Samath Dharmaratne, Farshad Pourmalek, Mehrdad Forouzanfar, and Nate Nair worked on running the earliest data through the earliest versions of the model. A number of experienced DisModers from previous Burden of Disease studies were invaluable as well, and thanks specifically to Mohsen Naghavi, Rafael Lozano, Steve Lim, Colin Mathers, Majid Ezzati, and Jan Barendregt. These experts brought in an army of new DisMod users, and thanks are due to all of them for their patience and perseverance in doing time-sensitive work with pre-alpha software.

Particular thanks to some who suffered the most: Jed Blore, Rosanna Norman, Saeid Shahraz, Maya Mascarenhas, and Gretchen Stevens. Jiaji Du joined early on as a software engineer, and his help, together with important software contributions from Brad Bell, made our unhardened research code strong enough to support the weight of the GBD 2010 project. Ben Althouse also made important contributions to the look and feel of the web app we used during those long days. Many additional thanks are due to Evan Laurie, Brad Bell, and Greg Anderson for taking on the task of updating the software implementation of the methods described here, which have already been used in the GBD 2013 project to much acclaim. Kelsey Pierce, Tasha Murphy, Patricia Kiyono, and Adrienne Chew were all instrumental in coordinating the process of turning scattered mathematical equations and PowerPoint slide decks into the edited volume you now hold. Finally, Hannah Peterson arrived as part of the IHME Post-Bachelor Fellowship at just the right time to provide a huge amount of assistance in completing a number of chapters for the first draft of this book.

ADF would also like to thank Jessi Berkelhammer and the rest of his family for their patience and support throughout the process of developing DisMod-MR and getting the methods all written down. The original timeline called for this book to be published before Sidney was born, but slipping deadlines and competing priorities delayed it until after Ida was one.

While we certainly could not have done this work alone, we bear full responsibility for any errors.

Introduction

Abraham D. Flaxman, Theo Vos, and Christopher J.L. Murray

This book, *An Integrative Metaregression Framework for Descriptive Epidemiology,* is a full-length treatment of new meta-analytic methods for descriptive epidemiology. From first principles, it develops the integrative systems model that constitutes the theoretical foundation of morbidity estimation in burden of disease studies like the Global Burden of Diseases, Injuries, and Risk Factors Study 2010 (GBD 2010). The estimation approach relies on producing age-specific prevalence estimates of the nonfatal outcomes of a vast array of diseases, injuries, and risk factors, for each country-sex-year.

The GBD 2010 study was a massive collaborative effort to measure levels and trends in all major diseases, injuries, and risk factors. Its first significant findings were published in a series of papers in December of 2012[1,2,3,4,5,6,7], which presented comprehensive sets of estimates of disease burden and attributable risk for 291 diseases and injuries and 67 risk factors, for 21 regions of the world, 20 age groups, and 187 countries. The author list for these papers contained 488 different researchers from 303 institutions in 50 countries.

As part of the GBD 2010 study, we developed a Bayesian metaregression tool specifically for synthesizing epidemiological data on nonfatal health outcomes This tool estimates a generalized negative-binomial model for all the epidemiological data with various types of fixed and random effects. These include age fixed effects, fixed effects for covariates that predict country variation in the quantity of interest, fixed effects that predict variation across studies due to attributes of the study protocols, and superregion, region, and country random intercepts. The tool uses Bayesian inference to estimate the parameters and sample from the joint posterior distribution of the model, incorporating all relevant descriptive epidemiological data. This approach is new, but the line of research builds on work in generic disease modeling that has been in use for almost 20 years in global health epidemiology.[8,9] However, until now, the descriptions of the models and the methods have been scattered throughout the scientific literature in a loose collection of journal articles, burden of disease reports, and operations manuals.

This book substantially extends the previous modeling efforts for years lived with disability (YLD) estimation in burden of disease estimation by formally connecting a system dynamics model of disease progression to a statistical model of the epidemiological rates measured in descriptive epidemiological research and collected in a systematic review. This combination of systems dynamics modeling and statistical modeling, which we call *integrative systems modeling,* allows the model to integrate all available relevant data. The statistical foundations for this approach fit into the broad framework of Bayesian methods, which we introduce briefly in Chapter 1. Because of the advanced numerical algorithms needed to fit these complex models, Chapter 8 provides some background on Markov chain Monte Carlo (MCMC) and other relevant computational methods.

Experience with the results of systematic review indicates that when all available relevant data are collected, they are often *sparse* and *noisy*. In GBD estimation, data sparsity often means that there are whole regions of the globe for which no data are available. The sparsity of data means that predictions of prevalence need to take advantage of relationships to risk factors and other explanatory variables in the metaregression, or else default to the average of a region, superregion, or the world. Dealing with noisy data is an additional challenge. In the regions or countries with multiple measurements, the results are often highly heterogeneous. The degree of heterogeneity is far beyond what is expected on the basis of sampling error and indicates considerable nonsampling variance. The sources of nonsampling variance include challenges in sample design; lack of a representative sample; and implementation issues in data collection, case definitions, and diagnostic technologies. To make matters more complicated, there is *true* geographic variation as well.

We will address a number of other common challenges in estimating the prevalence of nonfatal outcomes of disease:

- Based on biological or clinical knowledge, we may have strong prior beliefs on the age pattern of incidence or prevalence of a condition; for example, due to cumulative exposure to carcinogens, we expect the incidence of many cancers to increase with age, at least until some adult age. Another example is that the prevalence of bipolar disorder is zero in younger children.

- Published studies often use diverse age groups like 18–35 or 15 and older. For the GBD 2010 study, we needed to use data from different nonstandard age groups to generate coherent estimates for the 20 age groups in the study. Given that prevalence for most sequelae is strongly related to age, this issue is particularly important.

- For many conditions, the available studies use different case definitions. The review of diabetes prevalence studies identified 18 different case definitions in use. If all nonreference definition data are excluded, predictions can be based on only a limited number of studies. An alternative is to empirically adjust between different definitions using the overlap in available studies.

- Within regions or countries, the true prevalence for a sequela can vary enormously. The high level of hepatitis C infections in Egypt is an example in the Middle East and North Africa region. Such within-region heterogeneity in the true rates must be accommodated in a metaregression framework.

- Data are collected for many different outcomes, such as incidence, prevalence, remission, excess mortality, or cause-specific mortality. The mix of data varies across diseases and across regions for a disease. All these sources provide some relevant information for estimating prevalence.

The statistical model developed in this book focuses particularly on techniques for handling sparse, noisy data while also addressing these additional challenges. The book explores statistical models for overdispersed count data, covariate modeling to explain systematic variation in epidemiological data and to increase predictive accuracy for estimates where no data are available, and age pattern modeling to systematically incorporate expert knowledge about how epidemiological rates vary as a function of age. It also develops a theory of age-group modeling to address the heterogeneity in the specification of age groups that is commonly found during systematic review.

In the first half of this book, we present the theoretical foundations of integrative systems modeling of disease in populations. The second half of the book contains a series of applications of the model to the meta-analysis of a dozen different diseases.

An introductory example: smoking prevalence

To see how this new metaregression framework compares to, and extends, traditional meta-analysis, we begin with a simple example, a meta-analysis of smoking prevalence in the US for 2010. There were five nationally representative health surveys that measured smoking prevalence in this population, ranging from 16% to 25%. The forest plot in Figure 1 shows the measured values and precisions. A traditional fixed effect meta-analysis[10] would proceed by calculating the inverse variance weighted mean of the surveys, and predict a prevalence of 17.4% with 95% uncertainty interval (UI) of (17.3,17.6). But there is a problem with this approach: it appears to be more certain than is warranted. The uncertainty interval of the predicted prevalence does not overlap with the uncertainty interval of four of the five measured values.

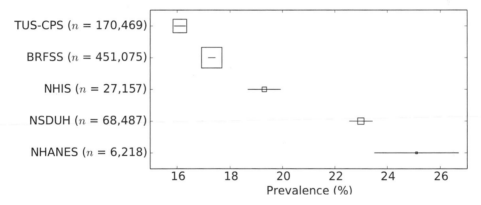

Figure 1. Data on smoking prevalence in the US for 2010 from five nationally representative health surveys.

The next step of complexity in a traditional meta-analysis is the introduction of the random effect model.[11] In this example, this approach produces a prediction with a different mean than the fixed effect model, and a much larger uncertainty interval. We will return to these traditional meta-analysis models in Chapter 1 and demonstrate how each is formalized as a simple model in the language of Bayesian statistics.

However, these traditional meta-analysis approaches fail to capture several important features of smoking prevalence that are of interest for burden of disease research and descriptive epidemiology in general. They do not capture the age-specific pattern of smoking prevalence, and they do not have a way to incorporate known differences between the studies (e.g., the National Health and Nutrition Examination Survey (NHANES) and National Health Interview Survey (NHIS) are conducted in person, while the Behavioral Risk Factor Surveillance System (BRFSS) and National Survey on Drug Use and Health (NSDUH) are telephone surveys, and the Tobacco Use Supplement to the Current Population Survey (TUS-CPS) is part telephone, part in-person).

In this example, there is great variation in the size of the surveys, and it is possible that the smallest of them (NHANES) is of lower quality for making a nationally representative estimate, simply due to stochastic variation. On the other hand, NHANES is an examination survey where the implementers go to great lengths to build up community support for their work and have higher response rates (77% for examined sample for all ages). NHANES also includes direct measurement of nicotine metabolites in the blood, which provides an alternative confirmation of the self-reported smoking prevalence measured by all the other surveys. This hints at the complex truth: there is much more to data source quality than simply sample size. Although meta-analysis provides some tools for integrating data sources of varying quality,[12] this can be a challenging area, and one where detailed work must proceed on a case-by-case basis.

We now turn to a more complete example, which demonstrates how the framework to be developed in this volume goes beyond traditional meta-analysis methods.

A motivating example: Parkinson's disease

As a motivating example, we now turn to the descriptive epidemiological metaregression of Parkinson's disease (PD). A systematic review of PD was conducted as part of the GBD 2010 study.[6] The results of this review needed to be combined to produce estimates of disease prevalence by region, age, sex, and year. These prevalence estimates were combined with disability weights to measure years lived with disability (YLDs), which were then combined with estimates of years of life lost (YLLs) to produce estimates of the burden of PD quantified in disability-adjusted life years (DALYs).

PD is a neurodegenerative disorder that includes symptoms of motor dysfunction, such as tremors and rigidity, in the early stages of the disease. As the disease develops, most patients also develop nonmotor symptoms, such as cognitive decline, dementia, and disordered sleep-wake regulation. The standard definition for PD diagnosis includes at least two of four cardinal signs—resting tremor, slowness in movements, rigidity, and postural abnormalities. There is no cure. Treatments slow the progression of the disease and alleviate some of the motor symptoms and disability.[13,14,15]

Systematic review for PD identifies 116 studies, yielding 782 data points by age and sex that met the inclusion criteria: 660 prevalence, 99 incidence, and 13 standardized mortality ratio (SMR) data points. It is instructive to consider each of these data types in detail.

Prevalence. Prevalence is the ratio of the number of individuals with the condition to the number of individuals in the population. This can be measured as a percent, but for rare conditions like PD it can be more appropriate to represent in other units, such as per 100,000. A typical example of a study found in the systematic review of PD prevalence is "Parkinson's disease in a Scottish city" by Mutch et al.[16] In this work, a research team used hospital records to screen for cases of PD in the city of Aberdeen between June 1983 and March 1984, and then interviewed and examined the individuals who screened positive, confirming 249 cases. Combining this with the 1981 census population of 151,616 living in the city, they reported a crude prevalence of 164 per 100,000. They also reported sex-specific measurements for five-year age groups, with prevalence peaking at 2,660 per 100,000 for men aged 85 and over.

The prevalence data collected in the PD systematic review exhibit many of the challenges listed in the beginning of this chapter and explored in detail in later chapters. They exhibit diverse age groups (Chapter 3), they include nationally representative studies and subnational studies, studies where cases were confirmed by a neurologist and studies by non-specialists, and studies with nonstandard diagnostic criteria (Chapter 6.1). The data span 36 different countries from 16 GBD regions, which may have true variation in PD prevalence levels (Chapter 6.4), and covariates such as smoking prevalence which are hypothesized to predict some of this variation (Chapter 6.2). It is very likely that within-country and between-study nonsampling variation are substantial (Chapter 2.5).

Incidence. Incidence is the rate at which people acquire the condition; it is measured per person per time unit. In the case of PD, it is appropriate to measure incidence units per 100,000 person years (PY). A typical study of PD incidence collected in systematic review is "Incidence of Parkinson disease and parkinsonism in three elderly populations of central Spain" by Benito-León et al. [17] In this study, researchers recruited a cohort of 5,160 subjects without PD and examined everyone they could find during three years of follow-up to identify the number of incident cases. The researchers found 30 incident cases of PD from this approach but could not evaluate 1,347 subjects. They assumed that the subjects lost to follow-up were missing at random and calculated a crude incidence of 236 per 100,000 PY with 95% confidence interval (CI) of 159 to 337. They also reported age- and sex-specific estimates with uncertainty quantified using 95% CIs, with incidence peaking at 1,017 per 100,000 PY for men aged 85 and over.

The incidence data collected in the PD systematic review exhibit all of the same challenges found in the prevalence data. Furthermore, the data are noisier because of the necessity of repeated examination and associated loss to follow-up. Not only does this make the measurements less accurate, it also makes incidence studies lengthier and more costly than prevalence studies. This may explain why systematic review identified over six times more data points for prevalence than for incidence.

Mortality. The standardized mortality ratio (SMR) is the ratio of the mortality rate of individuals with the condition to the mortality rate of the total population. Because it is a ratio, SMR is a unitless number. A typical study of PD SMR collected in systematic review is "A study of attitudes toward illness and its effect on mortality in patients with Parkinson's disease" by Kuroda et al. [18] In this study, researchers used health records to measure deaths among 433 patients with PD who received visits from a public health nurse between 1978 and 1987 in Osaka, Japan. This provided an average follow-up period of 4.1 years per patient and revealed 68 deaths, for a crude mortality rate of 38 per 1,000 PY. If PD cases had experienced the same mortality rates as the general population of Osaka over the same period, the expected number of deaths would have been 26.7, yielding an SMR of 2.54.

SMR data collected in the PD systematic review exhibit all of the challenges of incidence data. These data also require measuring the mortality rate of the general population, to use as the denominator in the standardization calculation. Although this quantity is often known much more precisely than the cause-specific mortality rate, even it can be a challenge in some settings. Furthermore, using it to standardize PD mortality assumes that the PD cases sampled have no elevated chance of mortality in addition to having PD; however, the sampling approach of convenience may lead to a nonrepresentative sample relative to the whole population, and this could bias the measurement of SMR.

A separate analysis of cause-specific mortality due to PD was carried out as part of GBD 2010, using the cause of death ensemble model (CODEm),[19] and provided 1,638 additional data points of cause-specific mortality rates (CSMRs) by region, age, and sex for the years 1990, 2005, and 2010. Cause-specific mortality is measured per person per unit time, and for a disease like PD it is convenient to use units of per 10,000 person years (PY). It is important to note that in this example, cause-specific mortality means that the decedent has died *from* PD (as the underlying cause of death) and not merely *with* it. This subtle distinction is elaborated on in Section 2.7 and demonstrated further in Chapter 20.

These sorts of CSMR data are themselves model-based estimates, which can be viewed as a limitation. The CODEm results are quite instrumental to the years of life lost (YLL) portion of DALY estimation, however, so when making prevalence estimates for DALY estimation, it is often not a problem to use these CSMR estimates as additional input data. There are cases where the prevalence of nonfatal health outcomes is used as a predictive covariate in CODEm, however, such as in modeling hepatitis C virus (HCV, see Chapter 13 for details). In this case, it would be circular to include CSMR estimates in the model that generates the prevalence estimates.

Data quality. As discussed above, there are inherent limitations to the different types of epidemiological data collected in systematic review, such as incidence measurements typically requiring repeated examination of individual subjects while prevalence measurements can usually be ascertained with a single examination. This is a data quality issue beyond the difference in sample size typically considered in analytic epidemiological meta-analysis. The quality of data sources may vary more than sample size among data of the same epidemiological type as well (e.g., prevalence data only), due to differences in study implementation, diagnostic criteria, or availability of diagnostic technology. Occasionally, there is enough information available to explicitly model this variation in study quality, which is the topic of Section 6.3, but this is not the case for the PD dataset.

Even when restricting the data to a specific geographic region, such as Western Europe, the data remain noisy and heterogeneous, as seen in Figure 2. Panel (a) of this figure shows a circle for each data point, where the position on the x-axis represents the jittered midpoint of the age group measured, and the position on the y-axis indicates the value of the measurement. Panels (b), (c), and (d) of this figure show a horizontal bar for each data point, where the left and right endpoints depict the start and end ages of the age interval measured, and the position of the bar on the y-axis indicates the value of the measurement. Section 5.1 describes our approach to making robust estimates in the face of such heterogeneous levels and overlapping age groups.

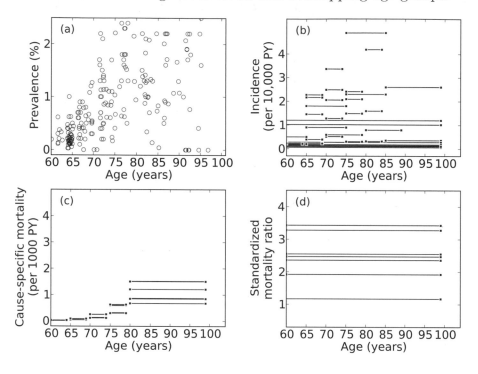

Figure 2. Data points from systematic review of descriptive epidemiology of Parkinson's disease, showing data from Western Europe on (a) prevalence, (b) incidence, (c) cause-specific mortality, and (d) standardized mortality ratio.

The data points represent the results of many different studies conducted for many different reasons. Some measured disease in a nationally representative sample population, while others were subnationally representative. Some relied on a diagnosis from a neurologist to measure existence of disease, while others allowed less expert opinion. Some used a nonstandard definition for PD, differing in some way from the gold-standard criteria. Study-level fixed effects, discussed in Chapter 6 and demonstrated further in Chapter 14, aid the model in explaining bias resulting from differing diagnostic criteria and study populations. The model finds no more bias associated with subnational studies than with national studies, estimating that the former are shifted in log-space by -0.03 on average, with a 95% uncertainty interval (UI) of $[-1.1, 1.2]$ (the precise meaning of the UI concept is given in Chapter 1). Similarly, the model estimates that studies that did not use a neurologist are shifted in log-space by 0.02 with a UI of $[-0.3, 0.3]$. Studies that used a nonstandard definition for PD diagnosis, on the other hand, were found to be systematically biased to lower levels of prevalence than studies using a standard definition. The effect coefficient for the shift in log-space was estimated to have a mean of -0.48 and a UI of $[-0.7, -0.2]$.

The totality of data collected in systematic review covers only 36 countries from 16 GBD regions, but GBD 2010 needed to include year-age-sex-specific estimates for 187 countries grouped into 21 regions. To predict year-age-sex estimates, explanatory covariates and fixed effects modeling provides a solution to the problem of missing epidemiological data, as developed in Chapter 6. The model for PD uses the amount of tea and coffee consumed per capita per day and national smoking prevalence as explanatory covariates. For an increase of one unit of tea/coffee intake per capita per day, the model estimates a shift in log-space of -0.34 with a UI of $[-0.5, -0.2]$. Similarly, for an increase of one unit in national smoking prevalence, the model predicts a shift in log-space of -0.02 with a UI of $[-0.05, -0.01]$.

Nonsampling variation that cannot be explained is another problem with such noisy and heterogeneous data. Chapter 6 explains how random effects can be used to estimate the systematic differences between countries within a region, regions within a superregion, and so on. Since this example contains data from Western Europe only, it is the country-level random effects that are relevant here. For example, the model estimates that prevalence in the Netherlands is above the regional mean, shifting estimates up by 20% (UI $[0, 50]$%). The model also estimates that prevalence in the United Kingdom is below the regional mean, shifting estimates down by 15% (UI $[0, 30]$%).

It is intuitive that there is a relationship between the different epidemiological parameters: every prevalent case was once an incident case, for example. Combining all parameters to produce internally consistent results is discussed in detail in Section 7.2. Through the process of data confrontation discussed in the following chapters, the meta-analysis produces a best estimate and uncertainty bounds of disease prevalence, as shown in Figure 3.

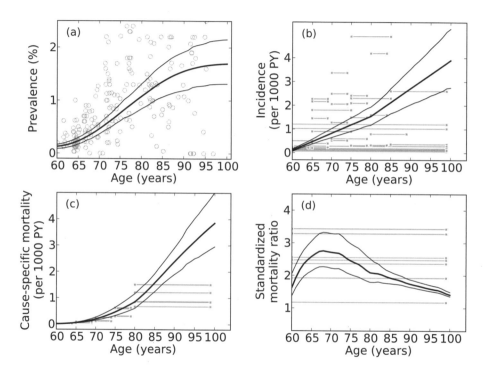

Figure 3. Estimates of age-specific rates of (a) prevalence, (b) incidence, (c) cause-specific mortality, and (d) standardized mortality ratio of Parkinson's disease in Western European females, 2005.

From systematic review to metaregression

To put the descriptive epidemiological metaregression framework developed in this book in its historical context, we will now provide a brief overview and introduction to meta-analysis and systematic review.

Meta-analysis combines the results of several studies that address a set of related research hypotheses. In its simplest form, this technique identifies a common measure of interest in all studies, for which a weighted average might be the output of the meta-analysis. For example, the weighting could be related to sample sizes within the individual studies.

The history of meta-analysis often begins with the work of Karl Pearson. In 1904, the British military commissioned Pearson to evaluate the military's typhoid inoculation campaigns.[20] Pearson obtained data on typhoid inoculation and mortality from two studies, one from India and one from South Africa, but determined that both sample sizes were too small to permit a reliable analysis. To increase the sample size, he combined the data and thus embarked on the first meta-analysis in public health. Unfortunately, this landmark study concluded little. With such heterogeneous data and irregular results, Pearson found it problematic assigning how much weight should be attributed to different results. Despite its inauspicious beginning, meta-analysis continued to develop.

The technique of systematic review has developed extensively since Pearson's time. The sheer number of publications every year has forced researchers to devise new ways to summarize and synthesize the torrent of results. From 1907, three years after the first meta-analysis, to 2007, the number of scientific publications has exploded. The number of abstracts compiled by the American Chemical Society has grown at 4.6% per year over that 100-year period. The number of publications compiled by the American Mathematical Society has grown at 5.9% per year. The number of publications in Compendex, a database of engineering studies, has grown at 3.9% per year.[21] PubMed, the largest database of biomedical literature in the world, now contains more than 21 million citations.[22] Despite this growth in publications, data are as heterogeneous and irregular as ever. This challenge certainly remains for data in descriptive epidemiology. Integrative systems modeling provides a framework to get the most information out of these disparate data.

As the number of scientific publications grew, identifying various sources to synthesize in a meta-analysis became a formidable task in its own right. This challenge led to the formalization of the process for identifying sources and to the development of systematic review. The Cochrane Collaboration is a group of over 28, 000 volunteers who review data from randomized controlled trials of health interventions.[23] In addition to the valuable information they provide on the efficacy of a wide range of interventions, they have created a detailed handbook for conducting systematic reviews. The Cochrane Collaboration defines "systematic review" as the methodic and explicit identification, selection, appraisal, collection, and analysis of relevant research. Meta-analysis then is defined as the use of statistical techniques to combine the results of studies from a systematic review.[24]

The Preferred Reporting Items for Systematic Reviews and Meta-analyses (PRISMA) group has also developed guidance for systematic reviews by standardizing the steps involved in a modern approach to the procedure.[25] PRISMA divides the systematic review process into four stages: Identification, Screening, Eligibility, and Included. In the Identification stage, the reviewer finds citations for studies by searching databases like PubMed and by contacting individual researchers and institutions. The reviewer uses a specific set of keywords for the database search in order to make that search transparent and replicable. In the Screening stage, the reviewer removes duplicated and unusable data. In the Eligibility stage, the reviewer excludes articles that do not match the explicit criteria for inclusion in the study. For instance, some systematic reviews in epidemiology only include evidence from randomized controlled trials and exclude observational data. In the Included stage, the reviewer finalizes the studies used for the systematic review.

Meta-analyses rely critically on the systematic review procedure. Here it is convenient to follow the terminology used by the Cochrane Collaboration and PRISMA and use "meta-analysis" to refer to statistical methods for combining evidence. This provides a clear separation between systematic review and meta-analysis and also divides meta-analysis from nonstatistical approaches of "research synthesis" or "evidence synthesis," such as combining information from qualitative studies.

As part of GBD 2010, groups of disease experts implemented this process for each disease and risk factor to be included. There are often data sources for descriptive epidemiology for which the measurements of interest have never been extracted and published, such as administrative databases of hospital admissions or regularly conducted health interview surveys, so the effort to capture data from unpublished sources was much more intense than in the traditional review of intervention studies in the Cochrane library. For some diseases, such as schistosomiasis, the vast majority of data obtained (more than 98%) came from studies that are not in the peer-reviewed literature. Regardless of the primary source of epidemiological measurements, the methodological challenge was then to take the results as input to generate estimates of epidemiological parameters of interest such as incidence, prevalence, and duration.

By far the most common use of meta-analytic techniques in epidemiology is to estimate the effect size of an intervention. By pooling all studies of the intervention effect, the meta-analysis provides a more precise estimate of effect size than that found in any individual single study.

The Cochrane guidelines caution not to compare studies with very different outcome measures of effect or very different patient populations when conducting a meta-analysis. [23] This is a subtle point and is more clearly developed in the meta-analysis of interventions than in the meta-analysis of descriptive epidemiological data. In fact, comparing studies with different outcome measures is at the heart of this book, which develops a method for comparing the results of descriptive epidemiological studies of disease prevalence, incidence, remission, and mortality risk that are focused on subpopulations from varying age groups, sexes, regions, and time periods.

Our framework is not without precedent, however. The next section discusses the legacy of "generic disease modeling," upon which our integrative approach to descriptive epidemiological metaregression builds.

History of generic disease modeling

Research into disease modeling for descriptive epidemiology has been accompanied by software packages since the 1990s. The development and refinement of these packages provides conveniently named milestones through the history of the approach. For example, DisMod I was software developed in the early 1990s to support analysis in the original Global Burden of Disease study. Computing power has increased dramatically over the 20-year period in which the DisMod family of generic disease modeling software has evolved, and the aspiration of methods has expanded as well. We will now trace how the approach has evolved from a simple spreadsheet model to a robust metaregression framework, which followed the timeline shown in Figure 4.

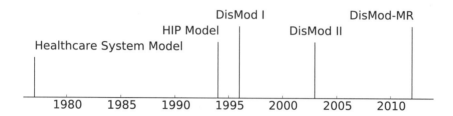

Figure 4. Timeline summarizing the succession of descriptive epidemiological modeling software from before the beginning of GBD studies until GBD 2010.

The precursor to the first DisMod software, the Harvard Incidence-Prevalence (HIP) Model, was a spreadsheet implemented in Lotus 123.[8] This model took as input a set of instantaneous incidence, remission, and excess mortality rates for five age groups and produced estimates of disease prevalence and duration. The model involved constructing a life table to simulate a cohort exposed to a set of age-specific incidence, remission, case fatality, and background mortality hazards. At each year in the life table, the model simulated a simple three-compartment model to provide estimates of the number susceptible, the number of cases, and the number of deaths to input into the life table for the next year. It was used primarily for three purposes: to find prevalence for conditions where incidence was known and reasonable assumptions about remission and excess mortality could be made; to find attributable deaths that were not directly coded to a specific cause; and to find incidence for conditions where prevalence was known. The third use required an interactive procedure in the HIP Model, since the input incidence was unknown.

As is often the case in science, a very similar approach had been developed previously by researchers at the International Institute for Applied Systems Analysis in Austria in the 1970s.[26] This work was part of a broad program to develop a generic Healthcare System Model to improve management and planning in the health sector. One component of this model was a computer program to estimate prevalence from incidence. That program evolved a population exposed to age-specific incidences of disease and death through time. Although it was designed specifically for terminal illness, it is similar to the DisMod line of models in many ways. It was applied to estimate the prevalence of malignant neoplasms in Austria, France, and Belgium.

Over the course of the first Global Burden of Disease Study, the HIP Model evolved into DisMod I.[27] This was formalized as a four-compartment model and a corresponding system of differential equations. As in the HIP Model, the input to DisMod I consisted of instantaneous rates for incidence, remission, and excess mortality, now specified for nine age groups. In addition, DisMod I was also used to estimate the average duration of disabling sequelae as a function of age. DisMod I was used iteratively by analysts working on GBD 1990 to identify a solution that matched the available data on prevalence, incidence, remission, excess mortality, and cause-specific mortality. DisMod I was used to address multiple challenges: mapping from incidence data to prevalence and vice versa, and assessing the consistency among incidence, prevalence, and cause-specific mortality.

DisMod II moved from forward simulation into the realm of optimization. It provided more control over inputs, as well as a graphical user interface and comprehensive user manual, making it more widely usable than previous iterations.[9] In addition to accepting input consisting of instantaneous rates for incidence, remission, and excess mortality, DisMod II was also capable of using age-specific prevalence and cause-specific mortality rates, as well as incidence as a population rate and duration. It also provided an algorithmic method for data confrontation wherein the downhill simplex method was used to minimize the weighted difference between the age-specific rate inputs and the output estimates of age-specific rates. Although DisMod II included the optimization, it was not framed as a statistical likelihood estimation.

The World Health Organization (WHO) distributed the DisMod II software without cost, and thus the generic disease modeling approach has been used widely in burden of disease studies over the last 10 years. These studies adopted the methodology of the global study but aimed to assess burden at a level of detail more relevant for national policymakers. At least 37 countries have undertaken national or subnational burden of disease studies, including Australia, Chile, Colombia, Malaysia, Mauritius, Mexico, Thailand, and Zimbabwe. [28,29,30,31,32,33,34,35]

Despite its wide application, DisMod II has been criticized. One methodological concern that emerged from extensive application of the model centered on the difficulty in producing consistent estimates that exhibited face validity—for example, age patterns that increased monotonically as a function of age. Despite strongly held prior beliefs on the part of domain experts, it was not uncommon for the prediction to show oscillations as a function of age, due to the contortions to which DisMod II would subject rates in order to produce consistent estimates as close to the single-rate-type input estimates as possible.

Another important challenge in the DisMod II work flow was the production of single best estimates for at least three independent rates to be used as input. Systematic review often finds multiple measurements of an age-specific rate, and only one could be the input to DisMod II. Transforming a large collection of measured values, often for incommensurate age intervals, to a single best estimate of disease prevalence was a difficult analytic challenge that was a necessary preprocessing step to do meta-analysis with DisMod II, often requiring an analyst to pick and choose the most appropriate data source for each parameter for each country-year rather than integrate all available data.

A third challenge with DisMod II was in producing robust estimates of parameter uncertainty. Although the system included a method to propagate uncertainty in the input parameters through to the output estimates, this was laborious and rarely used in practice.

Finally, although DisMod II excelled in providing consistent estimates from inconsistent estimates of several disease parameters for a single place and time, it was laborious for the data analyst to produce comparable estimates for a variety of different places and times. In the GBD 2010 study, there were 21 geographic regions to produce estimates for, at three different points in time, for males and females. Even an analysis that is trivial for one region/time/sex becomes burdensome when it must be replicated 126 times.

For GBD 2010, we completely redeveloped the method, continuing the trend toward including more formal inferential techniques in the estimation process.[6] The broad principle behind this approach is a form of nonlinear mixed effects modeling that we call integrative systems modeling (ISM) and can be characterized in two parts: a system dynamics model of process and a statistical model of data, considered together, so that instead of doing forward simulation, as is traditionally the case in system dynamics modeling, the model is used to solve an inverse problem. This method is emerging as a powerful approach for developing models that integrate all available data sources. On top of the compartmental model initially conceived for the HIP Model, we have layered an age-standardizing, negative-binomial, mixed-effects spline model, which is fitted directly to the data extracted in systematic review using Bayesian methods. The computational methods we used to fit this model also provide estimates of parameter uncertainty automatically, and, via a simple transformation, provide the 95% UI for all model estimates. We elaborate on this strength of our approach to Bayesian computation in Chapters 1 and 8.

This metaregression technique has been implemented in a free/libre open-source software package called DisMod-MR. The details of the approach constitute the bulk of the first part of this book. The second part is dedicated to a series of example applications, demonstrating all of the features developed in Part I.

What is not in this book

The development of this approach, its implementation in the DisMod-MR software, and its application in the GBD 2010 study are by no means the conclusion of this line of research. There is still much work to be done, and left to be considered further in the future are issues of computational efficiency, alternative approaches to spatial pooling, incorporating temporal trends more accurately, and the development of out-of-sample predictive validity measures using cross-validation (which raises again the issue of computational efficiency). We will return to these and other issues in more detail in Chapter 20 after developing the theory and providing example applications.

There are other important areas of inquiry in descriptive epidemiology that could benefit from the metaregression framework developed here, but which are not pursued in this volume. Estimates of inequality and differences in disease associated with race or with social or economic position have not been addressed here, although it would be possible to do so with appropriate data. Even sex-specific estimates, which were central to the GBD 2010 study, are not a topic of particular focus in this book. Although the general framework allows for time-trend analysis, the specific computational tools used in the GBD 2010 study dealt with this in a crude way only, and the examples in the second half of this book do not touch on it at all.

Nonetheless, there is plenty of material to present, and it is important to document the methods used in the GBD 2010 study, even if there are fruitful avenues for further development of the methods still open.

Part I

Theory and methods

Chapter 1

Background material on Bayesian methods

Abraham D. Flaxman

The phrase "Bayesian statistics" may have an intimidating sound to some. It evokes an air of controversy with others. For the purposes of this book, however, it is simply a method of convenience. The statistical approach pioneered by Laplace and Bayes in the 18th century turns out to be a flexible way to bring together different types of data to make estimates that incorporate all of the available information. The Bayesian way emerged as an approach to statistical inference in the 1950s and has grown to prominence in the last twenty years, due perhaps to efficient algorithms, faster computers, or simply a growing understanding of when it works well.[36] This chapter is not intended to provide a complete course in Bayesian methods, as several excellent books are wholly devoted to this topic.[37,38] Here I merely hope to introduce the concepts that will be used in the rest of this book. This may help some readers who have not worked extensively with this approach understand my motivation, and perhaps it will also help readers who have worked extensively with this approach understand my notation and perspective.

In the mathematical theory of probability, Bayes' law is a simple equation:

$$\mathbf{P}(A \mid B) = \frac{\mathbf{P}(B \mid A)\mathbf{P}(A)}{\mathbf{P}(B)}.$$

This is an identity that follows trivially from the definition of conditional probability, and as a student I did not understand why it deserved to have anyone's name attached to it. However, when this mathematics is applied to connect observations to theory, Bayes' law becomes the central assumption for a whole philosophy. Although the theory and history of this tendency make a fascinating topic, in this chapter I will provide only an operational overview of Bayesian methods.

The Bayesian philosophy, in its purest form, gives names to each part of this equation and often uses specific symbols to guide the familiar reader through the process. The denominator of the equation above is unknowable and unnecessary, and instead of A and B the statisticians prefer θ and X. Using the symbol $\propto$ to mean "is proportional to," the Bayesian way is summarized by the formula

$$\mathbf{p}(\theta \mid X) \propto \mathbf{p}(X \mid \theta)\mathbf{p}(\theta).$$

In this formula, $\mathbf{p}(X \mid \theta)$ is referred to as the *likelihood* and $\mathbf{p}(\theta)$ is called the prior. I have switched from writing $\mathbf{P}(\cdot)$ to $\mathbf{p}(\cdot)$ to emphasize that this is usually a statement about probability densities, but this is not important for our purposes. In this formulation, X represents the data and θ represents the parameters; both are typically multidimensional. The left-hand side of this equation is called the *posterior*, and the Bayesian way typically combines data, prior, and likelihood function to obtain summaries of the posterior density.

A simple example will help to clarify this, and we turn to one now, based on the five nationally representative measurements of adult smoking prevalence for the United States in 2010 which were described in the Introduction.

1.1   A meta-analysis example: smoking prevalence

In the discussion of fixed effect meta-analysis, I mentioned that one simple way to combine all of the measurements into a single estimate is to take a weighted average using weights proportional to the inverse variance of the measurements. A simple likelihood function accomplishes this in the Bayesian way and can be written as

$$X_i \sim \text{Normal}(\pi, s_i^2),$$

where X_i is the prevalence measured in study i, and s_i is the standard error of the measurement. This notation relies on a number of conventions, and to write this out precisely in terms of the Bayes formula above requires first knowing that $A \sim \mathcal{D}$ means that random variable A is distributed according to distribution $\mathcal{D}$, and then translating the above into the more explicit formula

$$\mathbf{p}(X_i \mid \pi) = \frac{1}{\sqrt{2\pi}s_i} \exp\left(\frac{(\pi - p_i)^2}{s_i^2}\right).$$

The final ingredient, implicit in the statement above, is the assumption that all X_i are independent, so that

$$\mathbf{p}(X \mid \pi) = \prod_{i=1}^{5} \mathbf{p}(X_i \mid \pi).$$

To be completely explicit here, it is worthwhile to also write out the data, X, which in this case is a table with 5 rows and 2 columns,

$$X = \begin{bmatrix} X_1 \\ X_2 \\ X_3 \\ X_4 \\ X_5 \end{bmatrix} = \begin{bmatrix} p_1 & s_1 \\ p_2 & s_2 \\ p_3 & s_3 \\ p_4 & s_4 \\ p_5 & s_5 \end{bmatrix} = \begin{bmatrix} 25.1 & 0.81 \\ 23.0 & 0.23 \\ 19.3 & 0.32 \\ 17.3 & 0.07 \\ 16.1 & 0.11 \end{bmatrix}$$

There is a school of statistics that stops here and uses the likelihood function alone to make inferences about model parameters (in this case π) from $\mathbf{p}(X \mid \pi)$. This approach relies on the *likelihood principle*, which hypothesizes that the value of π that maximizes the likelihood function is a good estimate of the true prevalence.

The Bayesian way requires one more ingredient beyond the likelihood function and the data, however, and that is the prior. Mathematically, this requires specifying a probability density for the model parameter vector θ (in this simple example θ has only one element, which I called π above). Any probability density can be used. For example, the uniform distribution on the interval $[5, 55]$, which would have the form

$$\mathbf{p}(\theta) = \begin{cases} \frac{1}{50}, & \text{if } 5 \leq \pi \leq 55; \\ 0, & \text{otherwise.} \end{cases}$$

The philosophical interpretation of Bayesian statistics ascribes much more importance to the choice of $\mathbf{p}(\theta)$ than this last paragraph suggests, however. In the subjective Bayesian tradition, this probability density is intended to encode the subjective belief about the model parameters *before* the statistician has seen the data (*a priori*, hence the name). However, it is not clear where these priors should come from, if individuals really have them a priori, and if they do, how to elicit them. A detailed discussion of this would certainly take us off our course, and it is left to the interested reader to pursue the more extensive texts on Bayesian analysis of data referenced above, or some of the more philosophical works on this challenging topic. [39,40,41]

Historically, there has been a focus on specific functional forms of priors that are convenient for computation in the pre-computer era. There are also some attempts to avoid the need for subjective priors, such as non-informative priors, diffuse priors, empirical priors, and weakly informative priors. From a pragmatic perspective, it is diffuse priors that I think show the most promise. This approach does not reject the subjective nature of the Bayesian philosophy, but instead urges the analyst to encode a minimal amount of information in the prior.

The informative prior would be designed by me, as the analyst (ideally in consultation with domain experts), to represent my subjective belief about smoking prevalence before I've seen the data. Unfortunately, I've seen the data, so now I have to think back to what I was like before I collected it all. I do not know many smokers these days, given the health-conscious nature of my field and my city, so I might have guessed low, one out of 10. But I also know that the US is not all like Seattle, and when I lived in Pittsburgh and people could smoke in bars I saw quite a lot more of it. So it wouldn't surprise me to learn than three out of 10 adults smoked in 2010. But everyone knows that smoking is bad for you, so seven out of ten, that would surprise me. The kernel of a density function that roughly captures this belief is the following:

$$\mathbf{p}(\pi) \propto \exp\left(\frac{(\pi - 10)^2}{(20)^2}\right).$$

This normal distribution also happens to be a convenient prior for hand calculation, because the functional form of the posterior will be easy to express when combining this prior with the likelihood above. It is a little bit weird, however, since it says that I have non-zero probability of finding a prevalence less than 0 or more than 1. The equations work, but the statistical philosopher (or applied epidemiologist) might prefer to truncate it into the following:

$$\mathbf{p}(\pi) \propto \begin{cases} \exp\left(\frac{(\pi-10)^2}{(20)^2}\right), & \text{if } 0 \leq \pi \leq 100 \\ 0, & \text{otherwise.} \end{cases}$$

An uninformative prior for this case could be to simply say that all values of π are equally likely a priori,

$$\mathbf{p}(\pi) \propto 1,$$

while a diffuse prior might look like the truncated normal distribution above, but with a much larger standard deviation, to indicate that while my best guess is 1 out of 10 smoke, nothing is off the table:

$$\mathbf{p}(\pi) \propto \begin{cases} \exp\left(\frac{(\pi-10)^2}{(1000)^2}\right), & \text{if } 0 \leq \pi \leq 100 \\ 0, & \text{otherwise.} \end{cases}$$

Finally, an empirical prior for this case would attempt to use the data in some simple way to come up with the prior, for example, calculating an unweighted mean of 20 and standard deviation of 3.8 from the five measured prevalences, and then using these parameters in a normal distribution:

$$\mathbf{p}(\pi) \propto \exp\left(\frac{(\pi-20)^2}{(3.8)^2}\right).$$

Although there can be a lot of fuss about these issues, in the present example, for many choices of priors, the resulting estimate of prevalence is not substantially different (and not very good). To see what difference these priors makes, however, it is necessary to spend a moment discussing what we will do with our posterior distribution once we have likelihood function, data, and prior all in hand.

Although Bayes' law is a fine definition of the posterior in terms of the likelihood, data, and prior, it is really summaries of the posterior distribution that are of practical interest. The mean of π under its posterior distribution, for example, is a convenient point estimate for the prevalence of smoking. It can be written as

$$\hat{\pi} = \int \pi \mathbf{p}(\pi \mid X) d\pi.$$

The median and mode of the distribution are also of interest, and it is reassuring when they are all similar values.

It is often of interest to know something about the spread of the posterior distribution, and one convention used in this book is to refer to the narrowest interval that contains 95% of the probability density as the 95% uncertainty interval (UI), or 95% highest-posterior density (HPD) interval, to be precise.

Table 1.1. Posterior distribution mean and spread for fixed effect meta-analysis with alternative prior distributions.

Prior	Posterior Mean	95% UI
Uniform$(5, 55)$	17.44	$(17.32, 17.55)$
Normal$(10, 20^2)$	17.44	$(17.33, 17.56)$
TruncatedNormal$_{[0,100]}(10, 20^2)$	17.44	$(17.32, 17.56)$
Uninformative	17.44	$(17.33, 17.55)$
TruncatedNormal$_{[0,100]}(10, 1000^2)$	17.44	$(17.33, 17.56)$
Normal$(20, (3.8)^2)$	17.44	$(17.32, 17.55)$

Finding the mean, median, mode, and UI of the posterior distribution for a complicated model is an area of active research, and some methods that make this possible are developed in detail in Chapter 8. For this example, however, the parameter space is one-dimensional, so it is possible to find all of these quantities with relatively simple calculations. The results are shown in Table 1.1.

One appealing approach to model checking is to compare observed data (or summary statistics thereof) to the *posterior predicted distribution* for the data. The idea here is that building the model requires specifying a likelihood for observed data, and this often can function as a generative distribution as well. Informally, we can augment the model above with

$$p_i^{\text{repl}} \sim \text{Normal}(\pi, s_i^2).$$

It is computationally very easy to implement this, although formally including this in the model is more of a challenge and is deferred to the texts referenced above.

This provides a way to critique the model: comparing the distribution p_i^{repl} to the observed value of p_i shows that the observed data are very unlikely accorded to the posterior predictive distribution.

1.2   Another meta-analysis example: random effect model of smoking prevalence

One problem with the model in the previous section is that the uncertainty interval of the predicted prevalence does not overlap with the uncertainty interval of four of the five measured values. The random effect model provides a way address this. It extends the model in the previous section to include an additional parameter that captures additional error in the measurements, beyond the sampling error included in the data. This can be accomplished by introducing a latent variable u_i for each observation, to represent the nonsampling error in each measurement, this can be written informally as

$$X_i \sim \pi + u_i + \text{Normal}(0, s_i^2),$$
$$u_i \sim \text{Normal}(0, \sigma^2).$$

One way to understand this model is that there is an unknown prevalence π for the whole population, and some different unknown prevalence for each of the measurements (due to nonsampling error) with value $\pi + u_i$. Although there is not an explicit explanation for this variation between measurements, the model is now flexible enough to represent sampling and nonsampling error.

This hierarchical formulation includes enough information to write out the complete likelihood function (from the first line), as well as some of the prior (from the second line), but does not describe the prior in full, which must also include π and σ somehow. Since each u_i and σ_i appear precisely once and always together, computationally it is not necessary to include u_i terms in the parameter vector θ, although theoretically there is nothing wrong with doing so, and in more complicated models, it can be the only way.

If we limit our attention to priors that treat σ and π independently, completing the model requires only specifying $\mathbf{p}(\sigma)$ and $\mathbf{p}(\pi)$. Now, however, the estimates of prevalence derived from the mean and spread of the marginal posterior distribution of π are more sensitive to the choices. Details about the computational methods necessary to obtain such estimates are deferred to Chapter 8. Table 1.2 shows how influential the changes in priors can be in this random effect meta-analysis case. Note the much wider uncertainty intervals in the random effect meta-analysis estimates, as compared to the fixed effect meta-analysis in Table 1.1.

Table 1.2. Posterior distribution mean and spread for random effect meta-analysis with alternative prior distributions. The uncertainty interval estimates are much wider than those from the fixed effect meta-analysis, and the posterior mean is higher as well.

Prior	Posterior Mean	95% UI
Uninformative	20.07	$(13, 26)$
Exponential(1)	20.09	$(16, 23)$
Normal$(1, 1^2)$	20.08	$(17, 22)$
Normal$(3.8, (3.8)^2)$	20.09	$(16, 23)$

1.3 Summary

This short introduction to Bayesian methods is not intended to provide a complete treatment of the subject, but I hope that it is helpful for some readers. The Bayesian model specifies a distribution for the likelihood and for the prior and then applies Bayes' law to go from data to posterior. As we shall see in future chapters, this approach is quite flexible and is capable of incorporating many elements that are useful in descriptive epidemiological metaregression.

Chapter 2

Statistical models for rates, ratios, and durations

Abraham D. Flaxman

A central decision when modeling epidemiological data with Bayesian methods is the choice of the data likelihood function. The particular functions that I consider for use as likelihoods when modeling descriptive epidemiological rate, ratio, and duration data are the topics of this chapter. These are what I call rate models, and they are precise, mathematical functions, intended to quantify how likely each data measurement is, for particular settings of the model parameters.

This is a statistical model of data and should not be confused with the models seen frequently in the tradition of mathematical epidemiology, where the focus is to produce a simple representation of the *process* of a disease. Each of the models in this chapter, whether we apply it to modeling rates, ratios, or durations, is simply an equation. The equation quantifies precisely how likely a certain data observation is for a given setting of the model parameters. This equation defines a likelihood function, which, as mentioned in Chapter 1, is the centerpiece to a whole school of statistical methods, based on the likelihood principle and maximum likelihood estimation. The likelihood function is also central to the Bayesian way, and Bayes' rule combines the likelihood and the prior to obtain the posterior. This chapter explores a range of alternative likelihood functions, any of which could be used for descriptive epidemiological metaregression. I often call them rate models for short, although they can be used for modeling ratios, durations, and even risk factor exposures, as well.

Before diving into these rate models, however, it is helpful to see where this piece fits into the metaregression model as a whole. A useful thought experiment to guide the development of a metaregression technique is to consider how the model would proceed if, for each and every study identified in systematic review, complete data were available for all subjects in the study (this is sometimes called microdata in survey research, or individual patient data (IPD) in meta-analysis). Of course, it is unusual that IPD are available for even *one* study from the systematic review in descriptive epidemiology. (Pooled analysis of IPD is more common in analytic epidemiology, for example the Asia Pacific Cohort Studies Collaboration and its meta-analysis of the effect of diabetes on the risks of cardiovascular disease.[42]) If all the IPD were available, say for all the prevalence studies conducted on schizophrenia (an example I will return to in the next section), modeling could proceed through standard techniques for analyzing binary data, such as logistic or probit regression, with fixed effects to explain some of the nonsampling variation, such as differing diagnostic criteria, and random effects to model the additional nonsampling variation, such as inherent differences between populations (if they exist).

Viewed in this light, the task of a metaregression model is to produce the results that would be obtained from an analysis of all the microdata, if they were available. The approach that will be developed below decomposes into three parts: the epidemiological rate model, which captures the sampling error in systematic review data; the age-interval model, which addresses the heterogeneity of age groups reported in the literature; and the covariate model, which models the nonsampling variation between different sources of data through fixed and random effects.

The key to connecting the data for different epidemiological parameters, such as incidence and prevalence, is the systems dynamics model presented in Chapter 7. This *model of process* describes how the *models of data* are related to each other. I will return to the model of process once the model of data is fully developed. The model of data is a statistical model that has its core features defined by its likelihood function. By *likelihood function*, I mean a probability density function that maps each possible parameter value to a non-negative number, conditional on the observed data values.

2.1 A motivating example: schizophrenia prevalence

To clarify the role of the likelihood function with an example, I turn now to the meta-analysis of population prevalence of schizophrenia in adult males. Strictly speaking, prevalence is a ratio, although in the literature the term "prevalence rate" is often used to mean prevalence ratio. The prevalence of a condition in a population is the ratio of individuals with the condition to all individuals in the population.

The forest plot in Figure 2.1 shows the results of combining 16 studies using seven different data models. As the figure demonstrates, the choice of data model can have a substantial effect on the estimated median, as well as on the uncertainty. The models I display produce point estimates ranging from 1.2 to 4.0 per $1,000$ person-years and uncertainty intervals with widths ranging from 0.1 to 2.9. When analyzing noisy data, the choice of the data model matters.

In what follows, I will develop a collection of data models, starting with the simplest and then increasing the complexity, while identifying the benefits and drawbacks of each. The models to come, in order, are

- the binomial model,

- the beta-binomial model,

- the Poisson model,

- the negative-binomial model,

- three variants of the normal model,

- the lower-bound data model.

2.2 Binomial model

Conceptually, the simplest model I consider for epidemiological data is built from the binomial random variable. Random variable X is *binomially distributed* if it has probability distribution

$$\mathbf{P}[X = k \mid n, \pi] = \binom{n}{k} \pi^k (1 - \pi)^{n-k}$$

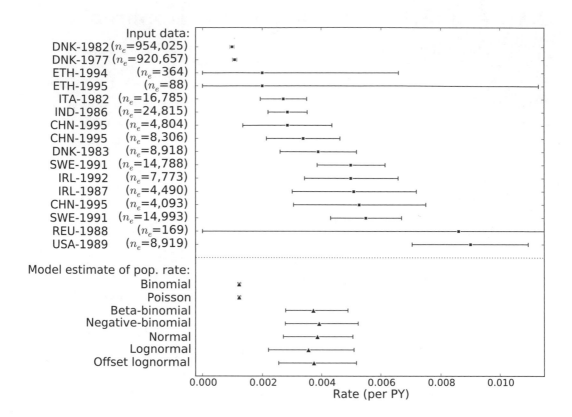

Figure 2.1. Forest plot summarizing seven alternative models for meta-analysis of adult male schizophrenia prevalence at the population level. The input data are labeled by the three-character country code and year of the study. The median estimates range from 0.0012 to 0.004 per person-years, and the width of the 95% uncertainty interval ranges from 0.1 to 2.9.

for some π with $0 \leq \pi \leq 1$. I have used Greek to emphasize that π is a model parameter, while n and k are data.

Although this equation may appear opaque, the intuition behind it is simple: n individuals were tested for a disease, and k tested positive. The formula then follows from the assumption that each individual tested positive with probability π, and that if I know π, then knowing about the test results of any subset of individuals gives me no information about the test results for the others (these events are "independent").

This description in the previous paragraph is particularly relevant to a study that measures the *prevalence* of a disease in a population. As mentioned above, prevalence is a *ratio*, not a rate. It is a unitless metric, often expressed as a fraction or a percentage. Incidence, remission, and mortality rates, on the other hand, are *rates*, measured per unit time. For example, incidence is often expressed in the units of "per person-year" or "per 1,000 person-years." Nonetheless, the binomial distribution can be the basis of a statistical model for rates as well as for prevalence. I will argue that it is not a very good model, and the fact that, in its intuitive description, it may have the wrong units is only one of its shortcomings. It is instructive to begin with simple models and make them more complicated until they are just complicated enough.

The binomial distribution inspires a computationally tractable data model for an observed population prevalence rate of r in a sample population of size n:

$$\mathbf{p}(r \mid \pi, n) \propto \pi^{\lfloor rn \rfloor}(1 - \pi)^{\lceil (1-r)n \rceil}.$$

Here $\mathbf{p}(\cdot)$ denotes a probability density function, $\lfloor \cdot \rfloor$ is the "floor" operator, which rounds real numbers down to the largest integer less than or equal to the operand, and $\lceil \cdot \rceil$ is the "ceiling" operator, which rounds up.

Note that it is not necessary to include the normalization term $\binom{n}{\lfloor nr \rfloor}$, because this does not depend on the model parameter π. This constant of proportionality is necessary to make this data model truly a probability density function for any π and n. But I will never need to know this constant, and I use the "proportional to" symbol $\propto$ instead of equality to emphasize this fact.

In terms of the thought experiment from the introduction, this model is equivalent to an analysis of all available microdata by fully pooling all individual measurements from all studies. It simply uses the sample population from each study together with the rate to find the number of positive observations. In the parlance of meta-analysis, this is a "fixed-effect meta-analysis," because the rate is modeled as fixed across all populations. [10]

One way to compare the posterior distribution to the available data is a graphical representation known as a funnel plot. The funnel plot was developed to identify publication bias in meta-analysis [43] and consists of a scatter plot where the measured value is compared to the standard error of the measurement. In my context of examining model fit, it is helpful to superimpose the posterior distribution on the same value-by-error axes.

The funnel plot in Figure 2.2 shows the posterior distribution of this rate model for $\pi = .004$. The handful of square markers show the observed rate (r)

and study size (n) from 16 studies of schizophrenia prevalence. The black line labeled "95% uncertainty" shows the region where the binomial rate model predicts that 95% of the observations will lie. This figure shows the potential problem with this model: the data gathered by systematic review are often much more dispersed than this distribution predicts. The binomial model row of the forest plot in Figure 2.1 shows the implications of this problem in the case of schizophrenia prevalence: two large studies are responsible for pulling the estimate below most of the observations, while the pooled uncertainty interval is so small that it does not overlap the uncertainty of most of the data points.

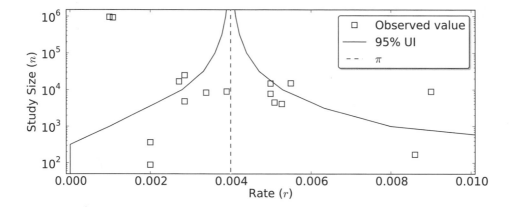

Figure 2.2. Funnel plot showing posterior distribution for the binomial rate model with $\pi = 0.004$ (95% uncertainty interval [UI] shown by black line), with data from systematic review for adult male schizophrenia prevalence overlaid for comparison (observations marked by squares).

There are two clear problems with this model—biased estimates and unreasonably high confidence when modeling noisy data. The model appears biased because many measurements are larger than the upper limit of the uncertainty interval, while none are smaller. The uncertainty interval appeared too small because it does not account sufficiently for noise in the measurement of r. If a study of $50,000$ people from subpopulation A finds prevalence of 2 per $1,000$ and a study of the same size in subpopulation B finds 6 per $1,000$, then the binomial model predicts that a third study conducted in subpopulation C will have prevalence of 4 per $1,000$, with an uncertainty interval of $[3, 5]$ per $1,000$ (I use the 95% highest posterior density [HPD] interval as the uncertainty). I have no problem with the point estimate; picking the mean of the two populations seems just right. But the uncertainty interval lacks face validity. It would be much more reasonable to have an uncertainty interval as large as, e.g., $[1, 7]$, instead of one as small as this.

Another way to quantify the mismatch between the binomial rate model and the observed data is through the posterior predictive check, an in-sample goodness-of-fit test that graphically compares the observed data to the posterior distribution for the data. Figure 2.3 shows $1,000$ draws from the posterior distribution for each of the data observations, together with the observation itself. The model predictions are compressed, showing a cloud of predicted points that often does not include the observation. Trusting the results of such a model leads to inappropriately high certainty about the nature of these noisy data.

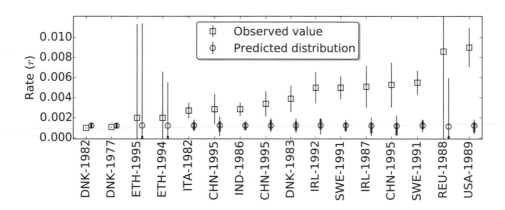

Figure 2.3. Posterior predictive check for binomial model fitted to adult male schizophrenia data. The input data are labeled by the three-character country code and year of the study on the x-axis. Circles and error bars show mean and 95% uncertainty interval for the posterior distribution of the binomial model, and squares show the observed data. The 95% confidence interval marked by error bars around each square shows the sampling error for each observation, based on the sample size alone. More than half of the data observations fall below the posterior distribution samples, indicating that the model is biased and not capturing the heterogeneity observed in the data.

2.3   Beta-binomial model

A theoretically appealing extension to the binomial model is the beta-binomial model.

Formally, a beta-binomial random variable X has the following probability distribution:

$$\mathbf{P}[X = k \mid n, \alpha, \beta] = \int_{\pi=0}^{1} \mathbf{p}(\pi \mid \alpha, \beta) \binom{n}{k} \pi^{k}(1-\pi)^{n-k}\mathbf{d}\pi,$$
$$\mathbf{p}(\pi \mid \alpha, \beta) \propto \pi^{\alpha-1}(1-\pi)^{\beta-1}.$$

The intuition behind this model is simpler than the equation. As in the binomial model, each individual tests positive for the condition independently with a probability π, but now π itself is not fixed across the population, but rather is a random variable, distributed according to a beta distribution with parameters α and β. The kernel of the beta distribution is given by

$$\mathbf{p}(\pi \mid \alpha, \beta) \propto \pi^{\alpha-1}(1-\pi)^{\beta-1}$$

and has a high degree of flexibility. It always takes values between 0 and 1, making it an appropriate distribution for a probability. Figure 2.4 shows the probability density of the beta distribution for several combinations of α and β.

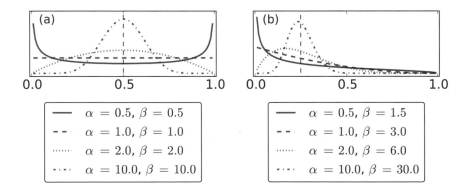

Figure 2.4. Probability density for the beta distribution for a range of α and β values. The dashed vertical line shows the expected value, which is one-half for all distributions in panel (a) and one-fourth for all in panel (b).

The beta-binomial distribution inspires the following data model for an observed rate of r in a population of size n:

$$\mathbf{p}(r \mid \alpha, \beta, n) \propto \int_{\pi=0}^{1} \pi^{\alpha-1}(1-\pi)^{\beta-1}\pi^{\lfloor rn \rfloor}(1-\pi)^{\lceil (1-r)n \rceil}\mathbf{d}\pi.$$

Although this equation may look imposing, it has a simple representation in terms of the binomial model in Section 2.2 and latent variables for each data point

$$X_i \mid \pi_i \sim \text{Binom}\left(\pi_i, n_i\right),$$
$$\pi_i \sim \text{Beta}(\alpha, \beta).$$

This model extends the binomial model in a way analogous to a random-effects model in traditional meta-analysis[10] (or in linear regression[44]). By introducing additional dimensions into the parameter space, the model is able to capture the dispersion beyond the binomial model that we see in funnel plots of real data. This can be interpreted as a model that recognizes that most studies are not identical and should not be completely pooled. Figure 2.5 shows the beta-binomial funnel plot, as well as the posterior predictive check for this model on the same data as used in Figure 2.3.

This model addresses the theoretical shortcoming raised in the previous section: if studies of $50,000$ people show prevalences of 2 and 6 per $1,000$, then the posterior distribution of the beta-binomial model has mean 4 with uncertainty interval $[1, 8]$, which seems quite reasonable.

2.4   Poisson model

There are two traditional approximations to the binomial distribution, depending on how large k is in relation to n. When k/n is large, the normal distribution is used, and when k/n is small, the binomial is similar to the Poisson distribution.

Since I expect disease prevalence to usually fall in a "small k/n" setting, I will not develop the normal model in detail now, although in Section 2.6 I will develop a model based on strictly increasing transformations of the normal distribution that include a normal model as a special case.

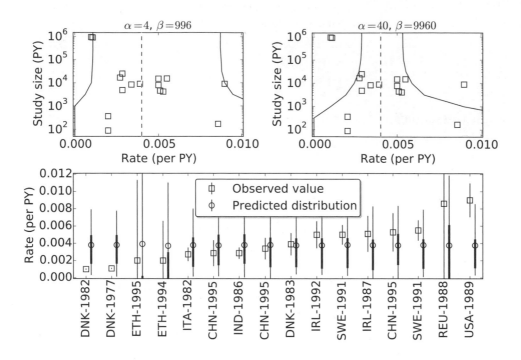

Figure 2.5. Funnel plots and posterior predictive check for the beta-binomial model. This model captures the heterogeneity in the observed data more faithfully than the binomial model from the previous section. However, the estimation procedure requires the introduction of a latent parameter for each data observation, and integrating out these latent variables is too computationally demanding to be feasible in many current applications.

The Poisson distribution is given by the equation

$$\mathbf{P}[X = k] = \frac{\lambda^k e^{-\lambda}}{k!},$$

and it can be understood intuitively as the number of times a "memoryless" event occurs in a unit time period. Setting $\lambda = \pi n$ produces an approximation to the binomial distribution that is quite accurate for large n and small k.

My Poisson rate model, which is defined from the Poisson distribution in a manner analogous to the way the binomial distribution was converted to a binomial rate model above, is the following:

$$\mathbf{p}(r \mid \pi, n) \propto (\pi n)^{\lfloor rn \rfloor} e^{-\pi n}.$$

It is also subject to all of the concerns raised about the binomial model. When modeling rates with nonsampling variation at the level typically found in systematic review, it will produce inappropriately low estimates of uncertainty.

There is one key benefit to this model compared to the binomial and beta-binomial models, however. The Poisson model assigns a nonzero likelihood to rates larger than 1. Although prevalence is always less than 1, it is theoretically possible to have incidence rates greater than 1 (per person-year), and remission rates are often greater than 1. For prevalence, which, as discussed above, is actually a unitless ratio of cases to population size, having nonzero probability of values greater than 1 is incorrect. But for incidence, remission, and excess mortality, which are measured per unit time, having a model with a natural interpretation in the same units is appealing.

2.5 Negative-binomial model

The negative-binomial model is a generalization of the Poisson model to allow for overdispersion. It provides a particularly appealing distribution for the likelihood. Its strange name comes from the formula that proves it sums to 1, and hence is a valid probability distribution:

$$\mathbf{P}[X = k \mid \lambda, \delta] = \frac{\Gamma(k + \delta)}{\Gamma(\delta)k!} \left(\frac{\delta}{\lambda + \delta}\right)^{\delta} \left(\frac{\lambda}{\lambda + \delta}\right)^{k}.$$

Unlike the beta-binomial distribution, this complex formula can be approximated accurately without numerical integration.

However, the closed-form expression for the likelihood obscures the intuition behind the negative-binomial distribution, which is quite similar to the intuition behind the beta-binomial distribution (but less clear from its name). Through a bit of algebra, the negative-binomial distribution can be represented as a hierarchical model where the observed data come from a Poisson distribution, and the parameter of the Poisson distribution is itself a random variable that comes from a gamma distribution:

$$X_i \mid \mu_i \sim \text{Poisson}(\mu_i),$$
$$\mu_i \sim \text{Gamma}(\lambda, \delta).$$

Here the gamma distribution is defined by

$$\mathbf{p}(\mu \mid \lambda, \delta) \propto \mu^{\delta-1} \exp\left(-\mu\delta/\lambda\right).$$

The identity

$$\frac{\Gamma(k+\delta)}{\Gamma(\delta)k!} \left(\frac{\delta}{\lambda+\delta}\right)^{\delta} \left(\frac{\lambda}{\lambda+\delta}\right)^{k} = C_{\lambda,\delta} \int_0^{\infty} \frac{e^{-\mu}\mu^k}{k!} \mu^{\delta-1} e^{-\mu\delta/\lambda} \mathbf{d}\mu$$

for an appropriate constant $C_{\lambda,\delta}$ verifies this interpretation.

Through this lens, the negative-binomial model can be seen as a natural adaptation of the traditional random effects model in linear regression to the Poisson case, where each observation comes from a different Poisson model and the Poisson parameters of these models are all drawn from a common gamma distribution.

In this parameterization, the δ parameter controls the overdispersion. When δ is large, the distribution is close to the Poisson from the previous section, and when δ is close to zero, the distribution diverges to an uninformative distribution on the non-negative integers. For intermediate values of δ, the distribution has variance that scales super-linearly with λ, according to the formula $\text{Var}[X] = \frac{\lambda(\delta+\lambda)}{\delta}$.

Thus, a rate model based on this distribution provides benefits in handling nonsampling variation similarly to the beta-binomial distribution but in a formulation that is much less demanding computationally. The negative-binomial rate model for observing a rate of r in a population of size n is

$$\mathbf{p}(r \mid \pi, \delta, n) \propto \frac{\Gamma(\lfloor rn \rfloor + \delta)}{\Gamma(\delta)} \left(\frac{\delta}{\pi n + \delta}\right)^{\delta} \left(\frac{\pi n}{\pi n + \delta}\right)^{\lfloor rn \rfloor}.$$

In this formulation, again, when δ is large, this reduces to the Poisson model. Now for δ near zero, it becomes an uninformative distribution on the rationals obtained by dividing the integers by n.

Figure 2.6 shows funnel plots for two levels of overdispersion, as well as the posterior distribution for the negative-binomial model.

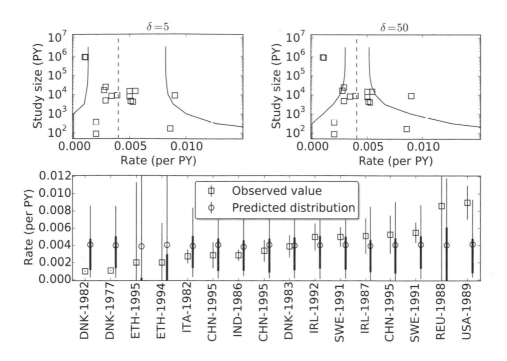

Figure 2.6. Funnel plots and posterior predictive check for the negative-binomial model. This model captures heterogeneity in observed data using an "overdispersion" parameter δ and can be interpreted as a hierarchical model, where each observation is drawn from a Poisson distribution that has its parameter drawn from a gamma distribution. When δ is very large, the negative-binomial model is equivalent to the Poisson model. The posterior predictive check shows that the uncertainty interval in the posterior predictions contains all the observed data, indicating that this model is sufficiently flexible to represent the observed heterogeneity.

2.6 Transformed normal models

Some epidemiological data are not related to count data at all. Duration studies and studies measuring the relative risk of mortality are two that come up frequently in systematic review. For duration data, a normal model is sufficient, and a lognormal model is appropriate for modeling relative risk data, which can be thought of as a ratio of count variables.

Transformed normal models have also been used for mortality rates in the past [45,46,47] and are worthy of continued consideration for modeling the incidence, prevalence, remission, and mortality as an alternative to the negative-binomial model.

In this section, I will develop a general transformed normal model and compare it to the negative-binomial model. The adjective "transformed" refers to a function that I will keep quite general for now, only requiring it to be strictly increasing and differentiable; that is, for any $x > y$ the transformation f must have $f(x) > f(y)$ and $f'(x)$ must be defined. Then the transformed normal model will be derived from the normal distribution, defined by the probability density kernel

$$\mathbf{p}(x \mid \pi, \sigma) \propto \frac{1}{\sigma} \exp\left\{ -\frac{(x - \pi)^2}{2\sigma^2} \right\}.$$

For any increasing, differentiable function f, this distribution can be converted to an f-transformed normal model with probability density

$$\mathbf{p}(r \mid \pi, \sigma, f, s) \propto \exp\left\{ -\frac{[f(r) - f(\pi)]^2}{2\left[(sf'(r))^2 + \sigma^2\right]} \right\},$$

where s is the standard error of the rate r, which is more convenient than the effective sample size n in this case. The denominator of the exponent deserves some additional discussion. For the identity function $f(x) = x$, the derivative $f'(x) = 1$, and the denominator simplifies to $2(s^2 + \sigma^2)$, a familiar "inverse variance" weighting, where σ is a random effect to account for overdispersion. When f is a more complicated function, the term $sf'(r)$ approximates the standard error of the transformed value $f(r)$. Although more sophisticated approximations are possible, experience dictates that the nonsampling variation (parametrized by σ) is always larger than the chance variation, so a simple approximation of the chance variation is sufficient.

Some common transformations of f used in related work yield the lognormal model $f(x) = \log x$, the logit model $f(x) = \text{logit}(x)$, and the probit model $f(x) = \text{probit}(x)$. All these approaches have a significant drawback, however. The transformation is not defined for $x = 0$, so these models cannot use data showing rates of zero. There are two common methods to fix this: dropping all zeros and adding a small offset. Dropping measurements of zero is clearly problematic, as it leads to systematic bias in the data that remain and produces estimates larger than the truth. This is especially problematic for high-quality studies that focus on the age pattern of a disease, where it is quite reasonable for some age groups to have zero cases observed. The effect of dropping zero is to overestimate the rates in these age groups.

Adding a small offset, such as 0.5, is an alternative solution, and indeed, this is the approach taken for cause-specific mortality estimation in a similar approach to mortality modeling.[45] In some settings the choice of offset can be guided by considerations of the noise floor of the measurements, or by a pseudo-counts argument based on Bayesian prior considerations. The selection of the offset is often ad hoc, however.

Within the framework of the transformed normal model, there is room to put the solution on firm theoretical foundations. For example, by taking $f_\zeta(x) = \log(x + \zeta)$, I obtain the "offset log-transformed model," which does allow rates of 0, simply by taking a positive value for ζ. This model will not be used extensively in the example application to come later in this book, but it seems like a promising approach. It is particularly appealing in the way it decomposes the sampling variation into an additive error ζ and a multiplicative error σ, and I expect that it will prove useful in the future. For completeness, here is the probability density for the offset log-transformed model:

$$\mathbf{p}(r \mid \pi, \sigma, \zeta, s) \propto \exp\left\{ -\frac{[\log(r + \zeta) - \log(\pi + \zeta)]^2}{2\left[\left(\frac{s}{r+\zeta}\right)^2 + \sigma^2\right]} \right\}.$$

Figure 2.7 shows funnel plots for two levels of overdispersion, as well as the posterior distribution for the offset lognormal model.

2.7 Lower-bound data model

When I develop the integrative systems model (ISM) of disease in a population in Chapter 7, cause-specific mortality rate (CSMR) data will often constitute a special case, to be handled differently from all other epidemiological rate data. These CSMR data come from careful processing of large numbers of vital registration system outputs, from verbal autopsy studies, and from some other sources. But when I introduce the compartmental model of disease in a population in Chapter 7, there will be an important distinction about where CSMR data fit in. Unlike incidence, prevalence, and remission data, they do

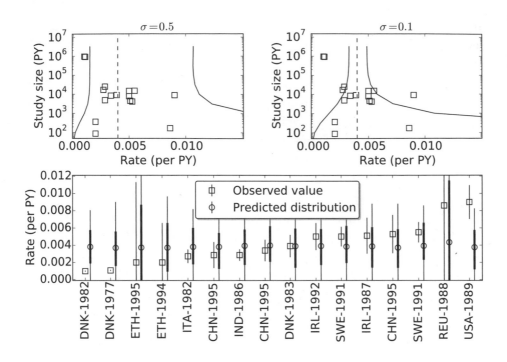

Figure 2.7. Funnel plots and posterior predictive check for the offset lognormal model. This model captures heterogeneity in observed data using a dispersion parameter σ and also includes an offset parameter ζ that interpolates between lognormal and normal models.

not correspond directly to any rate in the compartmental model. But unlike standardized mortality rate, relative risk, and duration data, they cannot be derived as a function of compartmental model parameters, either. This is because of the operational requirement in vital registration systems that each death have a single underlying cause. The excess mortality rate in the system dynamics model from Chapter 7 is not entirely compatible with this idea.

It is unfortunate that the development of this data model comes before the development of the ISM in Chapter 7, and if the reader finds it unclear on first reading, I hope it will make more sense after exposure to the material in the later chapter. It seems worthwhile to group all of the rate model material together, despite the resulting out-of-sequence conceptual dependency.

The theoretically grounded way to develop the lower-bound data model is based on an extension of the compartmental model from Section 7.2 to include CSMR data explicitly simply by splitting the excess-mortality hazard h_f flowing out of the with-condition compartment C into two parts (see Figure 20.2). These parts, $h_{f'}$ and $h_{f''}$, would sum to h_f. The quantity $h_{f'}$ would denote the portion of excess mortality caused directly by the disease, so any individuals that exit compartment C via the flow with hazard $h_{f'}$ would have this condition listed as the underlying cause of death on their death certificate. The quantity $h_{f''} = h_f - h_{f'}$ would then denote the "excess excess mortality," which is to say the elevated mortality among individuals dying *with* the condition but not *of* the condition.

Proceeding down this path with the proposed terminology promises to be extremely confusing! It is also a challenge because the data available have never been sufficient to separately estimate $h_{f'}$ and $h_{f''}$ with much accuracy. When the model is more flexible than the data, it is hard to fit and the results are hard to interpret.

This motivates the alternative approach that I have taken, which implicitly separates excess mortality into $h_{f'}$ and $h_{f''}$ but does not try to explicitly represent both in the model. It is a "lower-bound" likelihood, which contributes nothing to the likelihood as long as the observation is less than the prediction, and uses the Poisson rate model when the observation is above the predicted level:

$$\mathbf{p}(r \mid \pi, n) \propto \begin{cases} (\pi n)^{\lfloor rn \rfloor} e^{-\pi n}, & \text{if } \pi < r; \\ 0, & \text{otherwise.} \end{cases}$$

Chapter 20 provides an example application of this.

2.8 Quantification of uncertainty

The quantification of uncertainty in metaregression is worthy of special attention. The binomial, beta-binomial, Poisson, and negative-binomial models developed above all rely on a quantification of uncertainty in terms of persons or person-years, denoted by n. This is a stylized notion, however, based on a simple model of the data-generation process that uses a simple random sample. In systematic review, it is common to find more complex survey designs, and more sophisticated quantification of uncertainty is often reported. I call the corresponding n the "effective sample size," because it denotes the size that the sample would be if an identically powered study *did* use simple random sampling.

The transformed normal models above require a quantification of uncertainty in terms of standard error, denoted by s. Many studies collected in systematic review report this value directly, but many others do not.

It is useful to have a simple set of conversions to translate between the n needed for the count models, the standard error needed for the transformed normal models, and the often-reported 95% confidence interval, which does not appear directly in any of the rate models above. The approximate relationships between these quantities are standard, and developing more precise transformations is not justified due to the large amount of nonsampling variation in systematic review data.

To represent a standard error s in terms of a 95% confidence interval (a, b), I have used the normal approximation

$$s = \frac{b - a}{2 \cdot 1.96}.$$

To represent an effective sample size n in terms of a standard error s and a observed rate r, I have two options. For prevalence data, where the standard error is for a ratio and hence constrained to be between 0 and 1, I have used the binomial approximation

$$n = \frac{r(1 - r)}{s^2}.$$

For other epidemiological rates, such as incidence and remission rates, where the standard error is for a rate that is nonnegative but could potentially be larger than 1, I prefer the Poisson approximation

$$n = \frac{r}{s^2}.$$

Some studies from systematic review report point estimates for age-specific rates but quantify uncertainty only at coarser levels of aggregation, for example, the sample size of the entire study. In these cases, I recommend a rough approximation that splits the n for the entire population among the subpopulations proportionally to the population age structure.

Surprising as it may be, some studies from systematic review do not report quantification of uncertainty at all. It may be acceptable to exclude these studies, and this exclusion criterion should ideally be articulated at the beginning of the systematic review process. Sometimes data are so sparse that it is not feasible to exclude studies that do not quantify uncertainty, however. In this case, I recommend imputing the missing uncertainty interval (UI) values by taking them to have UI width equal to the 90th percentile value of the UI widths from the observations that do quantify uncertainty.

2.9 Comparison

Making a quantitative comparison of the models at this point is challenging. A simulation study depends critically on the distribution used to simulate the data sets. Choosing a simulation distribution that matches the assumptions of any model will yield results that make the chosen model look superior. A comparison based on out-of-sample predictive accuracy would be preferable, but disease data are so sparse and noisy that such a comparison could be meaningless, especially without including the adjustments for covariate effects and age integration, which are developed in the next two chapters. A handful of diseases have data homogeneous enough in age and geography to attempt a comparison of the models, but these are necessarily special cases, and extending such findings to other settings must be done with caution. On the other hand, something is better than nothing.

To this end, I compared all models using a holdout cross-validation approach. I used the Markov chain Monte Carlo approach, described in Chapter 8, to generate 1,000 samples of the model parameters from the joint posterior distribution for each model, using random subsets of the data on schizophrenia prevalence and on epilepsy prevalence collected from systematic review[6] in the model likelihood. The schizophrenia dataset is familiar from earlier in this chapter and contains only 16 observations. The epilepsy dataset contains many more rows of data, with 1,719 observed prevalence values, and the level appears to vary little as a function of age, time, or geography. I included each observation in the subset to fit independently with probability 0.75, yielding a subset with 8 rows expected for schizophrenia and around 1,300 observations for epilepsy. Then I fitted each model with this subset and used the fit to predict values for the observations that were not included in the subset. For 100 replicates, I measured the bias, median absolute error, coverage probability, and computation time for each model. The results are shown in Table 2.1.

Table 2.1. Mean results of holdout cross-validation of rate models for 100 replicates for out-of-sample prediction, ordered by increasing median absolute error (MAE).

Schizophrenia data:

Rate Model	Bias (pp)	MAE (pp)	PC (%)	Time (s)
Beta-binomial	0.08	0.08	94.6	213
Negative-binomial	0.00	0.16	96.5	76
Normal	0.01	0.17	94.3	63
Offset lognormal	0.01	0.17	92.7	84
Lognormal	−0.06	0.19	98.1	73
Binomial	0.28	0.25	11.4	49
Poisson	0.28	0.25	11.4	49

Epilepsy data:

Rate Model	Bias (pp)	MAE (pp)	PC (%)	Time (s)
Beta-binomial	0.33	0.26	29.8	182299
Negative-binomial	0.09	0.36	88.5	190
Normal	0.00	0.42	95.1	105
Offset lognormal	0.00	0.42	95.1	130
Lognormal	0.25	0.27	88.5	124
Binomial	0.38	0.26	3.2	101
Poisson	0.38	0.26	3.2	83

Note: Bias is the mean of observed minus predicted measured in percentage points (pp), median absolute error (MAE) is the median of the absolute difference between observed and predicted, probability of coverage (PC) is the fraction of observed falling within 95% uncertainty interval of prediction, and time is the computation time.

For the schizophrenia data, the beta-binomial model has the lowest median absolute error (MAE), but takes the longest to run, while the negative-binomial, normal, offset lognormal and lognormal models all have slightly higher MAE, and similarly low bias and accurate calibration. The binomial and Poisson models have substantially more bias, as well as higher MAE and lower probability of coverage (PC).

For the epilepsy data, the beta-binomial model has coverage probability 10 times higher than the binomial and Poisson models, which also minimize median absolute error, but takes 1,000 times longer to compute and is still far from the target probability of coverage of 95%. The lognormal model has the superior balance of MAE and PC, but cannot cope with data measurements of zero prevalence. All of these four models have substantial bias as well. In addition to being theoretically justified, the negative-binomial model has a balance of low MAE and high PC, with much lower bias. The normal and offset lognormal models have even lower bias and are perfectly calibrated, but have the highest MAE.

2.10 Summary and future work

This chapter has developed seven alternative rate models, all with benefits and drawbacks. The binomial model is simple and theoretically appealing but does not handle nonsampling variation, producing overconfident estimates in the face of noisy data. The beta-binomial model deals with overdispersion through a theoretically appealing extension to the binomial model, but it is too computationally demanding to use in my applications. The Poisson model is a close approximation to the binomial model and has all the drawbacks except that it can handle rates greater than 1, which is important for modeling remission rates. So it is the negative-binomial model, which extends the Poisson model analogously to the way the beta-binomial model extends the binomial model, that I prefer on theoretical grounds. This is the model that I have used for most of the applications to follow, where it is applied to represent data for incidence, prevalence, remission, excess mortality, and cause-specific mortality. It is not as amenable to analysis as I would like, however, and sometimes benefits from diffuse priors on the overdispersion parameter, an undesirable feature that slows down analysis by requiring sensitivity analysis. Transformed normal models are a promising alternative approach, and I have used the normal model for duration data in some of the following examples, as well as the lognormal model for standardized mortality rate data and relative mortality risk data. The offset log-transformed model seems particularly promising as an alternative to the negative-binomial model, and understanding its statistical and computational characteristics is a promising direction for future research. Like the negative-binomial model, however, the convergence of these transformed normal models also benefits from diffuse priors, a topic that deserves additional attention in the future.

Chapter 3

Age pattern models

Abraham D. Flaxman

The rate models of data in the previous chapter need several extensions to be truly useful in descriptive epidemiological metaregression. The most important is representing the differences in rates as a function of age. In this chapter, I develop the mathematical and statistical theory behind a model for age specificity in prevalence rates as well as other epidemiological hazard functions, such as incidence, remission, without-condition mortality, and excess-mortality hazards.

The unfortunate truth is that no one lives forever. Furthermore, the profile of disease changes dramatically as we age, with a set of diseases most troublesome in childhood that are nearly no problem in old age, and a completely different set that are unheard of in youth causing substantial burden among the elderly.

This chapter is concerned with representing age variability in disease models. The central idea in this chapter that that, although there may be great change between disease parameters from age 20 to age 80, the difference between age 20 and age 21 is generally not great. In more mathematical terms, the disease rates vary *continuously* as a function of age. The continuum has been an important area of study in mathematics, and many surprises lurk in the corners of any attempt to make it completely rigorous. However, for our purposes, it is enough to consider a particular class of continuous functions, called spline models. This term apparently comes from shipbuilding, and has the important related jargon of *knots*, which control the shape of the spline and where it may vary least smoothly. All of this is getting a little bit complicated, so let us proceed to some examples and develop things a step at a time.

Figure 3.1 shows age-specific all-cause mortality rates for five-year age groups. These mortality estimates are for females in Southern sub-Saharan Africa in 1990. A striking feature of this plot is the range of variation in mortality levels as a function of age. They vary by 850-fold between the minimum in the 10- to 14-year-old age group and the maximum at the oldest ages. Epidemiological rates also vary among regions, times, and sexes. A figure like Figure 3.1 for the high-income Asia Pacific region in 1990 would look very different, as would the Southern sub-Saharan Africa region in 2010. However, systematic variation as a function of *age* is often the largest source of variation by orders of magnitude, and furthermore, this variation is often distinctly nonlinear.

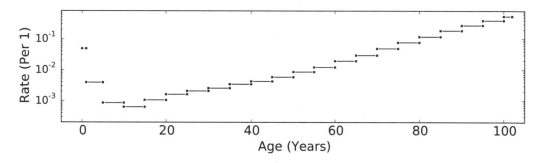

Figure 3.1. All-cause mortality for females in the Southern sub-Saharan Africa region in 1990 as a function of age shows the range of variation in age-specific rates. All-cause mortality is as low as 6 per $10,000$ PY at age 10 but rises above $5,000$ per $10,000$ PY at age 100.

The approach that I have taken for modeling age-specific hazards draws on the mathematical theory of spline interpolation and on the statistical theory of penalized spline regression. In nautical engineering, the term "spline" refers to a drafting technique used to design the curved hulls of ships in the days long before computer-aided design. In modern statistical practice, spline models are often used in time series analysis, where they represent the continuous variation in time of a variable of interest.

The mathematics necessary to use splines in descriptive epidemiological metaregression are developed in this chapter.

3.1   Definition of spline models

For my purposes, a spline model can be any piecewise polynomial function. Often I will require this function to be continuous, but not always. This is a departure from the conventions of statistical spline modeling, which focuses on continuous and continuously differentiable splines.[48,49]

I represent a spline model for an age-specific hazard $h(a)$ by a set of knots $a_1, \ldots, a_K$ and a set of piecewise polynomial basis functions $\{p_1, \ldots, p_{K'}\}$. Each knot has a corresponding basis function, and for higher-order splines, there may be additional basis functions as well, so $K \leq K'$. The model then has K' parameters, $\gamma_1, \ldots, \gamma_{K'}$, and takes the form

$$h(a) = \sum_{k=1}^{K'} \gamma_k p_k(a).$$

The mathematical definition of the model is straightforward, but the detail of selecting the piecewise polynomials remains to be developed. This is where the spirit of spline modeling resides. The knots $a_1, \ldots, a_K$ partition the age range into intervals. If I make each piecewise polynomial $p_k(a)$ equal to 1 on its interval (i.e., when $a_k \leq a < a_{k+1}$) and 0 otherwise, this yields a piecewise constant spline model. This is an important specialization, the simplest of my spline models. Using the notation $\mathbf{1}[a_k \leq a < a_{k+1}]$ to denote the function

$$p_k(a) = \begin{cases} 1, & \text{if } a_k \leq a < a_{k+1}; \\ 0, & \text{otherwise}; \end{cases}$$

and the convention that $a_{K+1} = \infty$, I can write out the piecewise constant spline model as

$$h(a) = \sum_{k=1}^{K} \gamma_k \mathbf{1}[a_k \leq a < a_{k+1}].$$

By taking the piecewise polynomial corresponding to each knot as 0 before its knot and a linearly increasing function after, the model specializes to a piecewise linear spline model, a continuous function that has a constant derivative at all nonknots. By adding an additional basis function that is not associated with a knot, this piecewise linear spline model becomes a flexible approximation for any nonlinear function and is the main form I have used in representing age-specific hazards in the work to come. I can write out the piecewise constant specialization of the spline model as

$$h(a) = \gamma_0 + \sum_{k=1}^{K} \gamma_k(a - a_k)\mathbf{1}[a \geq a_k].$$

I find that in applications of this model it is useful to represent the piecewise linear spline in an alternative basis, where the model parameter γ_k represents the values of $\log h(a_k)$ instead of the change in the slope at this point. This yields a more complicated set of basis functions, but it is not necessary to write out the basis functions explicitly.

Figure 3.2 shows the results of fitting spline models for age-specific hazards to simulated data to minimize the sum of the square differences between the predicted and observed values. When the piecewise constant model is fitted, it produces an age-specific hazard function consisting of a series of horizontal (constant) lines in each of the intervals between knots. Interval k has γ_k equal to the mean value of the simulated data between knots a_k and a_{k+1}, which is quite a sensible choice.

A more favorable and flexible fit to the data is achieved by the piecewise linear spline model, which produces a continuous function of age as its prediction. In many cases, a piecewise linear fit of this type is sufficient to capture the nonlinearity in the data, and this will be the typical model for epidemiological rates in the second half of this book. It is possible to go further along this path of smoothing, however, and splines that have continuous derivatives and even continuous second derivatives are popular alternatives, achievable by simply choosing different piecewise polynomials for the basis functions.

3.2   Choosing knots

To this point, I have taken as given the number and location of the knots in the spline model. However, selecting the number and location of the knots is an important task, and can influence the model results substantially.

When data are abundant and age patterns are clear, models will not be very sensitive to the choice of knots, but when data are not abundant, or when the age patterns are not clear from the data, knot selection is a delicate part of the modeling process. In this setting, knot locations should be chosen a priori, based on the anticipated age groups available in the data as well as the anticipated changes in the epidemiology of disease being modeled as a

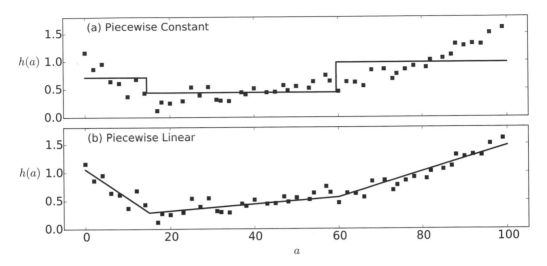

Figure 3.2. Spline interpolation of simulated data. The true age-specific rate is piecewise log-linear, so none of the splines can represent it perfectly. The true age-specific rate and the models all have knot set $\{0, 15, 60, 100\}$.

function of age. For example, in a recent study looking at global trends in mean systolic blood pressure as a function of age, the modelers chose to use a cubic regression spline with knots located at ages 30 and 60.[50] These choices reflect the expectation, based on literature and prior knowledge, that the behavior of mean systolic blood pressure as a function of age would be distinct in these intervals due to low blood pressure in young adults and to survivor effects in elderly populations. As another example, Chapter 10 uses premenstrual syndrome to examine the effects of incorporating biological knowledge into the model as priors.

The approach of using expert knowledge to select the number and location of knots is a practical choice, but it is certainly not the only approach. Much literature is devoted to the choice of knot locations and the number of knots. An important direction for future work is to remove the reliance on expert knowledge to inform knot selection. This could proceed through model selection or model averaging of models with a variety of knot locations,[51] through techniques developed in the adaptive regression spline literature[52] or more mathematical approaches,[53] or by leaving spline models altogether and using Gaussian processes or some similar nonparametric model for the age pattern.[54,55]

3.3   Penalized spline models

One approach to address the challenge of knot selection is to include many knots in the model and then also include a penalty function to discourage the model from using the additional knots when the data do not call for them. This penalized spline model can be formulated in a Bayesian framework by introducing a prior that represents the belief that, in the absence of evidence, the age pattern does not vary. Mathematically, I have formulated this as a penalty on the root mean square of the derivative of the age-specific rate $h(a)$:

$$\left[\int_{a=a_1}^{a_K} \|h'(a)\|^2 \mathbf{d}w(a) \right]^{1/2} \sim N(0, \sigma^2).$$

This introduces an additional model parameter, σ, which can be viewed as a hyperprior and controls the amount of smoothing that the penalty creates.

For the piecewise linear penalized splines that will be used most frequently in the second half of this book, the derivative of h is constant between knots, so, with equal weighting for smoothing at all ages, the integral above simplifies to the following:

$$\int_{a=a_1}^{a_K} \|h'(a)\|^2 \mathbf{d}a = \sum_{k=1}^{K-1} \left[\frac{h(a_{k+1}) - h(a_k)}{a_{k+1} - a_k} \right]^2 (a_{k+1} - a_k)$$

$$= \sum_{k=1}^{K-1} \frac{[h(a_{k+1}) - h(a_k)]^2}{(a_{k+1} - a_k)}.$$

Figure 3.3 shows the effect of increasing the smoothing parameter σ when many more knots than necessary have been included in the model. Without smoothing, including many knots leads to estimates that are overly imprecise and wiggly. Smoothing, in the form of a quadratic penalty on the derivative of the age pattern, allows many knots to be included. But too much smoothing, for example, $\sigma = 0.005$ in this case, results in a model that does not reflect true patterns in the data.

3.4   Augmenting the spline model

There are a few ways to augment the spline model that are useful when modeling age-specific rates. Since the epidemiological rates I have modeled are

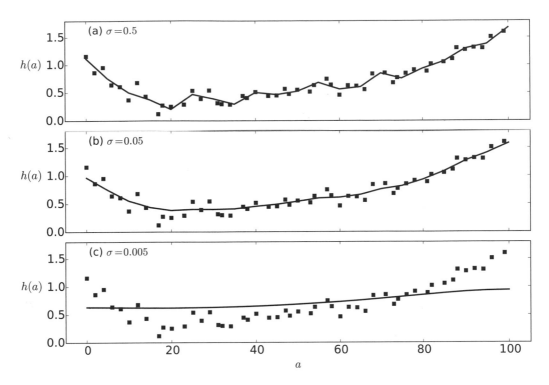

Figure 3.3. Penalized splines with an appropriate smoothing parameter σ reduces the challenge of choosing a set of knots to choosing a single smoothing parameter.

always nonnegative, I have parametrized the spline in terms of the log of the knot values, so that $h(a)$ is a piecewise linear spline model with knots $a_1, \ldots, a_K$, and

$$h(a_k) = c^{\gamma_k}.$$

To fit the model in a Bayesian framework, I have defaulted to giving these γ_i's diffuse priors (as described in Chapter 1),

$$\gamma_i \sim \text{Normal}\left(0, 10^2\right).$$

This has very little effect on the posterior distribution but makes the prior "proper" and also helps with algorithm convergence in some instances. Where relevant expert knowledge is available, I can replace this with a more informative prior (this idea is elaborated in Chapter 4).

Finally, to deal with the order-of-magnitude differences of age-specific rates, I have applied the smoothing penalty to the logarithm of the rate rather than to the rate itself. This creates an additional complication, however, because the informative priors often say that rates are 0 for certain ages. To avoid a situation where the smoothing penalty includes the log of zero, I have rounded up any γ_i values that are below 10 times the mean rate. The approach is operationalized as a penalty term in the prior:

$$\widetilde{\|h'\|} = \sqrt{\sum_{k=1}^{K-1} \frac{[\max(\gamma_k, \gamma_{\min}) - \max(\gamma_{k+1}, \gamma_{\min})]^2}{(a_{k+1} - a_k)(a_K - a_1)}} \sim \text{Normal}(0, \sigma^2),$$

where

$$\gamma_{\min} = \log\left[\left(\sum_{i=0}^{K} e^{\gamma_i}/10\right)/K\right].$$

The result of this unusual rounded-up penalty is to allow the age-pattern, as parameterized in log-space, to vary non-smoothly in relative terms for rates that are less than 10 times the average value. For example, in the Parkinson's disease example in the Introduction, the smoothing penalty is not applied to the estimates at very young ages, when there is almost zero prevalence of the disease.

3.5   Summary and future work

Taken all together then, the model for an age-specific hazard function that will be used in this book is

$$h(a) = \sum_{k=1}^{K-1} \mathbf{1}[a_k \le a < a_{k+1}] \left(\frac{a - a_k}{a_{k+1} - a_k} e^{\gamma_k} + \frac{a_{k+1} - a}{a_{k+1} - a_k} e^{\gamma_{k+1}} \right),$$

$$\gamma_k \sim \text{Normal}\left(0, 10^2\right),$$

$$\widetilde{\|h'\|} \sim \text{Normal}(0, \sigma^2).$$

The value of σ is a model parameter that will receive a very informative hyperprior: "slightly smooth" is represented by $\sigma = 0.5$, "moderately smooth" is represented by $\sigma = 0.05$, and "very smooth" is represented by $\sigma = 0.005$.

A limitation of this approach is that the modeler must make a selection of the number of knots, location of knots, and level of smoothing, and developing computationally feasible alternatives that rely on the data alone is an important direction for future work.

There are at least two alternative approaches to this: moving these parameters into the model or systematically comparing multiple models. It seems particularly challenging to fit models with the number of knots as parameters, and even models with a fixed number of knots are hard to fit when the knot locations are model parameters. Models with the level of smoothing as a parameter are possible to fit with moderate additional computation time, however, and with sufficiently informative data on age patterns, this is a viable approach.

Systematically comparing multiple models, for example a range of models with different numbers of knots and different knot positions, could be a more computationally feasible approach, although it requires choosing an appropriate metric of comparison. Although there are model comparison criteria such as Bayesian Information Criteria and Divergence Information Criteria, which are specifically designed for Bayesian modeling, using some form of hold-out cross validation seems to be emerging as the gold-standard approach, if computation time permits.

It is not necessary to choose a single best model from a range. A promising direction for future work is in so-called "ensemble models," which incorporate predictions from multiple models, appropriately weighted based on the predictive validity of each model.

The penalized spline approach may also be worthy of additional attention. Instead of using the rounded-up approach, switching over to an offset term inside the log would bring a pleasing symmetry to this and the offset log-normal model from the previous chapter. However, there is an extensive theory of smoothing splines and penalized splines that might provide even more appealing options.[49,53]

Chapter 4

Expert priors on age patterns

Abraham D. Flaxman

It is sometimes necessary to include additional expert knowledge on the age pattern of epidemiological rates. For example, data sparsity can take the form of a lack of information about age-specific hazards of disease in children. In diseases that are rare or nonexistent in children, the fact that incidence is effectively zero before a certain age is known by disease experts but not represented in the data collected by systematic review. The integration of this knowledge into the age-specific rate model from the previous chapter is quite straightforward and can be formulated in the Bayesian way as part of the prior distribution. This is where the somewhat opaque term "expert priors" comes from: it is simply a collection of additional factors multiplied into the prior distribution.

A benefit of the Bayesian methods that will be used to fit these models is the conceptual and practical simplicity of adding additional information to the age pattern model. This is implemented by choosing a more informative prior distribution. For example, if the epidemiology of a disease is such that the incidence level must be zero before age a_k, this can be incorporated by replacing the diffuse prior by the conditional probability density with this constraint included.

Three classes of additional information will come up frequently in the applications later in this book: level bound priors, level value priors, and monotonicity priors. This section describes how each can be implemented as an informative prior on the age pattern model.

4.1   Priors on level

A prior on the level value for certain ages says precisely that the age pattern should have that value for those ages. For example, Figure 4.1 shows the effects of adding a prior where the age-specific hazard function takes values extremely close to 0.1, 0.5, or 1.0 from age 0 to 15.

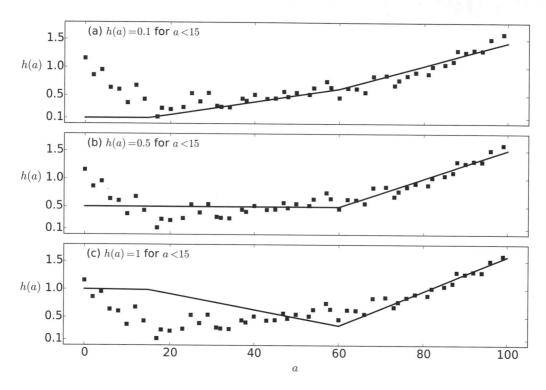

Figure 4.1. An informative prior on the level of $h(a)$ for interval $0 \leq a < 15$ changes the estimated rate dramatically for a between 20 and 60 and even leads to different estimates for $a = 100$.

These priors are implemented as "hard-soft constraints." For a value v on age range (a_0, a_1), the value of the spline model is replaced with the level value for the age range (which I call a hard constraint), and the prior density on the spline is augmented with a penalty term for the offset log difference between the level value of the unconstrained spline and v (which I call a soft constraint). The offset-log-difference penalty has the form

$$\log\left(h(a) + \epsilon\right) \sim \mathrm{Normal}\left(\log\left(v + \epsilon\right), \sigma^2\right),$$

where $h(a)$ is the age-specific hazard function, $\epsilon = 10^{-6}$ is the offset to avoid taking the log of 0, and $\sigma = 0.01$ is the magnitude of the penalty. In Bayesian terms, this encodes the belief that the spline is expected to be within 1% of the expert level value, provided the level value is not too close to 0.

A similar sort of expert knowledge on the plausible bounds on level is also useful, both in modeling noisy data and in increasing the numerical stability of estimation algorithms. Figure 4.2 shows the effects of three different upper bounds on the spline estimation from the same dataset as the previous figure.

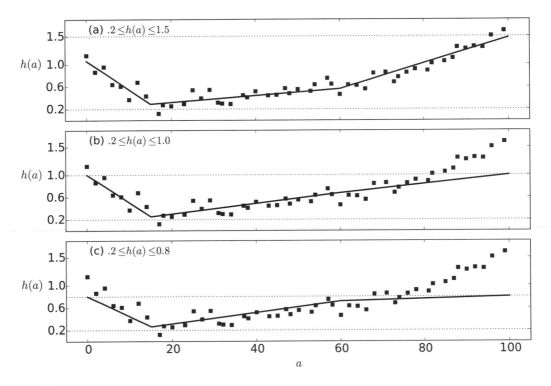

Figure 4.2. An informative prior on the upper and lower bounds of the age-specific hazard function $h(a)$ changes the estimated hazard function dramatically for ages where the data are outside the bounds. For ages where the data are inside the bounds, the estimates are also affected, but to a lesser degree.

Like the level value prior, this prior is also implemented as a hard-soft constraint. If the level bounds are $\ell_0 \leq h(a) \leq \ell_1$, there is a hard constraint that replaces the spline with a clipped version, $h^c(a) = \min\{\max[h(a), \ell_0], \ell_1\}$, and also a soft constraint that ensures that the original spline is close to the clipped spline in offset log-transformed space.

4.2   Priors on monotonicity

One common expert prior on age patterns is a strong belief that the function is increasing or decreasing over a certain age range. Mathematically speaking, these are priors on the sign of the derivative of the age pattern. For example, these priors can be implemented efficiently in Bayesian Markov chain Monte Carlo (MCMC) computation by conditioning on the differences of the age-specific hazard function $h(a)$:

$$h(a) \geq h(a+1) \text{ for } a : a_s < a < a_e.$$

The results of using such a prior are shown in Figure 4.3. When the prior is contrary to the data, the estimate will be as close to the data as possible while respecting the prior. For example, the age-specific hazard function in Figure 4.3c is the result of a prior belief that the age pattern increases from age 0 to 50 when confronted with data that clearly decrease over this age range.

For computational efficiency, the increasing and decreasing constraints are implemented as soft constraints. For a constraint that the function is decreasing between a_s and a_e, I include the following penalty term in the log-posterior:

$$-\epsilon \left[\sum_{a=a_s}^{a_e-1} \max\left(h(a) - h(a+1), 0\right) \right]^2$$

for $\epsilon = 10^{12}$. Comparing the function values on a single-year age grid (where $h(a)$ is compared to $h(a+1)$) relies on the spline knots all being at least one year apart. This approach also explains why the upper limit of the sum is $a_e - 1$.

An area for future work comes from another common expert belief: that the age pattern is unimodal. This is conceptually clear, but computationally it has proven more difficult to realize than monotonicity. While the monotonicity constraint maintains log-concavity of the posterior distribution (if it was log-concave to start with), a straightforward implementation of a unimodality constraint will result in non-log-concave posterior distribution, even if everything else is well behaved. This suggests that the difficulty in fitting such models is inherent in the local step method of the MCMC algorithms I

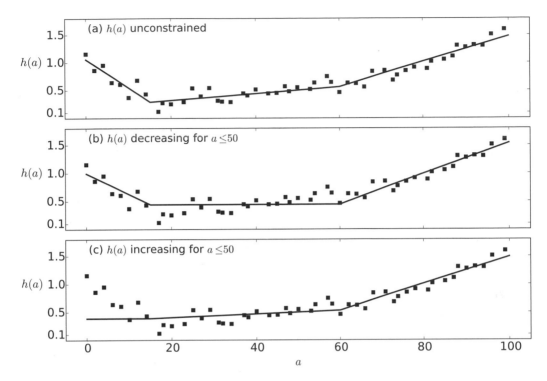

Figure 4.3. The expert belief that the age pattern is increasing or decreasing across an age range can also be implemented as a Bayesian prior.

have been using. Perhaps an alternative approach such as Hamiltonian Monte Carlo step methods or the population Monte Carlo algorithm would be more successful.[56,57,58] Alternatively, there are some approximations of the uni-modality constraint that may be easier to optimize over.[59]

4.3 Priors are not just for splines

Until now, all of the age patterns have been described as spline models, h_a. The compartmental model in Section 7.2 will substantially expand the age pattern with many derived quantities such as the age-specific prevalence and the relative mortality risk. These quantities are derived in Chapter 7. All three of the expert priors developed in this chapter are applicable to any age-specific function derived from the compartmental model. Most important, the age-specific prevalence can be augmented with expert priors on level values (e.g., birth prevalence is 0), level bounds (e.g., no population has prevalence above 10%), and monotonicity constraints (e.g., prevalence is increasing as a function of age). Relative mortality risk is another derived quantity for which experts often have strong priors.

However, this sort of modeling requires care. The system dynamics model enforces a precise consistency between the different epidemiological rates, and making strong assumptions about one will have implications for others. Sometimes these implications are counterintuitive.

As a practical matter, I recommend that modeling begin with as few assumptions about the level and slope of the age pattern as possible, after which expert priors may be added one at a time. The benefit of this is threefold. First, fitting the model without all the available expert knowledge allows the data to speak. If the estimates confirm the expert belief, that is reassuring, and if they show the opposite, that is interesting. Second, the MCMC algorithm has a pitfall: *nonconvergence*. A quick way into this pit is introducing inconsistent expert priors, for example, decreasing prevalence and prevalence of zero at age 0. By adding in expert priors one at a time, any inconsistencies that caused nonconvergence will be more easily identified. Third, it is essential to conduct a sensitivity analysis to understand how influential modeling assumptions are on the results. The gradual addition of expert priors will provide a starting point for this sensitivity analysis, showing which expert priors are essential to obtaining reasonable results and which are not as critical.

4.4   Hierarchical similarity priors on age patterns

There is one additional type of level prior worthy of a separate exposition. It is the one that I have used to implement the empirical Bayes approach described in Section 8.7. A discussion of the relative merits of the empirical Bayes approach[38] will be deferred for that section, but in short, I view this as a computational convenience that permits decomposing estimation of globally heterogeneous age patterns into subcomputations that can be run in parallel.

For GBD 2010, countries were grouped into 21 mutually exclusive and collectively exhaustive "regions" based on demographic and epidemiological similarity, as listed in Appendix . It is not necessarily the case that the age pattern of a disease is common across regions (Chapter 11 shows how the age pattern of pancreatitis varies even between countries in the same region).

In order to borrow strength between regions, it is therefore necessary to have a notion of similarity between age patterns. The simplest way to do this is to include a penalty on deviations of certain ages in the age-specific hazard model, for example

$$h(a) \sim \text{Normal}\left(\boldsymbol{\mu}_{\text{prior}}(a), \boldsymbol{\sigma}^2_{\text{prior}}(a)\right) \text{ for } a \in A.$$

Since the model must cope with the order-of-magnitude differences of age-specific rates, I have found it more robust to use an empirical prior relating the offset log-transformed rates:

$$\log\left(h(a) + \epsilon\right) \sim \text{Normal}\left(\log\left(\boldsymbol{\mu}_{\text{prior}}(a) + \epsilon\right), \left(\frac{\boldsymbol{\sigma}_{\text{prior}}(a) + \epsilon}{\boldsymbol{\mu}_{\text{prior}}(a) + \epsilon}\right)^2\right) \text{ for } a \in A.$$

This approach is crude, however, and leaves much room for further work. Although it succeeds at borrowing strength between regions in a way that allows for different age patterns, it is sensitive to the choice of ϵ and also to the set of ages A where the penalty is calculated. A promising direction for future work would be including the age-correlation structure in the model as well.

4.5 Summary and future work

This chapter has introduced and demonstrated the effects of level value priors, level bound priors, and monotonicity priors, all of which can be applied to the spline models from Chapter 3, as well as the age-specific rates that will be derived from the compartmental model in Chapter 7. However, these model assumptions must be justified, and future work is necessary in developing methods and procedures for conducting comprehensive sensitivity analyses and guaranteeing that the results are not unduly influenced by the choice of priors.

The application of empirical priors for age patterns is another area where future work will be important. There are alternative formulations for translating the estimates from a global model into priors for a regional model, such as a multivariate normal distribution with an empirically derived variance-covariance matrix. It remains to be seen if these more complex priors provide enough benefit to justify their use.

A prior related to the monotonicity priors which may be called a unimodality prior has often been requested during this work. Although it is straightforward to formulate the mathematical requirement that an age-specific hazard function have a single local maximum, all naive implementations have proven challenging for MCMC optimization. Developing a computationally tractable unimodality prior is an additional direction for future work.

Chapter 5

Statistical models for heterogeneous age groups

Abraham D. Flaxman

With a full development of statistical rate models for a single age group behind us, and the mathematical model for an age-specific rate function laid out as well, this chapter turns to a peculiar feature of population rate metaregression: the wide variety of age groups reported in the literature.

Age subgroup analysis is a common feature of epidemiological analysis, and refers to how the estimates of the epidemiological parameters measured are grouped by age. The broadest age groups come from sources like case notifications, where the entire population of a country forms the denominator and events occurring among all ages are reported together in a single number. On the other end of the spectrum, when studying mortality rates from a complete vital registration system it is possible to consider age groups of under a year, for example age 0 to 28 days for neonatal conditions, or age 0 to 24 hours for early neonatal conditions. Studies often stratify by five-year or ten-year age groups as well, but many studies use alternative age grouping based on idiosyncratic considerations such as local school ages or drinking laws. This chapter is devoted to developing and comparing a collection of statistical models that can integrate data on a heterogeneous set of age groups.

A typical example of the heterogeneity in age groups is shown for the systematic review results on atrial fibrillation (AF) prevalence[6] Figure 5.1. The midpoint of the age group is scattered against the width of the age group. Simply put, there is no standard set of age groups for AF research, and different studies report results with different age groups. Unfortunately, this phenomenon is far from unique to AF.

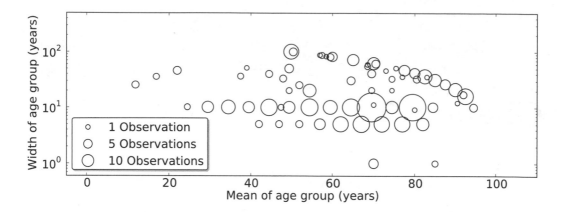

Figure 5.1. Mean and spread of age groups in the prevalence data collected from a systematic review of atrial fibrillation. The size of the circle shows how many observations of this age group were found in systematic review. There were 586 rows of prevalence data extracted, but the most common age group accounted for only 68 rows.

This variation in reporting would not be problematic if it were possible to access to the microdata from all the systematic review studies. For example, using microdata from a national health information system or from a demographic household survey, it would be possible to tally the prevalence rates by single-year age groups. Although each individual rate gathered in this way would have high variability, the rate model from Chapter 2 combined with the spline model for an age-specific hazard function from Chapter 3 would work together to produce an estimate that is as uncertain as it should be.

Although reanalysis from microdata is occasionally implemented in a GBD study, it is often not an option. I expect microdata reanalysis to become more frequent in national and subnational settings. In the more common situation where rate microdata are not available, the rates cannot be retallied into homogeneous age groups, and an alternative approach is needed.

This setting is in some ways similar to the settings where interval regression methods are applied in econometrics.[60,61,62] However, I have more information about the structure of the data that I can leverage in my model. I have considered several statistical approaches, and they will be compared and contrasted in this chapter. Before getting into the details, however, it is worthwhile to examine theoretically the way that age-grouping functions. I begin with a simple mechanistic model of the age-grouping process. A study conducts some sort of measurement on a population of individuals who are all of different ages, and then the epidemiological rate or rates of interest are tallied for age groups selected in some context-dependent manner. If the study was a prevalence study using a full census sample, for example, and if I use r_{a_0,a_1} to denote the rate for age group (a_0, a_1) and n_{a_0,a_1} to denote the subpopulation size of age group (a_0, a_1), then the identity

$$n_{a_0,a_2} = n_{a_0,a_1} + n_{a_1,a_2}.$$

says nothing more complicated than that the size of the subpopulation of age at least a_0 and less than a_2 is the sum of the size of the subpopulation between ages a_0 and a_1 and the size of the subpopulation between ages a_1 and a_2. Applying the same observation to the parts of these subpopulations that have the condition of interest yields the following identity:

$$r_{a_0,a_2} = r_{a_0,a_1} \frac{n_{a_0,a_1}}{n_{a_0,a_2}} + r_{a_1,a_2} \frac{n_{a_1,a_2}}{n_{a_0,a_2}}.$$

In a limiting case of a very large population with very fine age intervals, this becomes

$$r_{a_0,a_2} = \int_{a=a_0}^{a_2} r_{a,a+\mathbf{d}a} \frac{n_{a,a+\mathbf{d}a}}{n_{a_0,a_2}} \mathbf{d}a.$$

Undoubtedly, all real studies are more complicated than this full census of prevalence, but this is a starting point for conceptualizing where age-grouped rates come from. Roughly, they are integrals over instantaneous rates for infinitesimal age groups.

5.1   Overlapping age-group data

The primary way I like to display overlapping age-group data is with horizontal lines on a plot of age versus rate value, as shown in Figure 5.2. The level of the bars shows the rate value, while the width of the bars shows the range of ages included in the age group. It is often informative to augment these lines with error bars that show the uncertainty reported for each rate value, but for this section I have left out the representation of uncertainty to keep the plots as simple as possible.

Each of the horizontal lines in Figure 5.2 can be represented as a triple (a_s, a_e, r), where a_s is the starting age of the age group, a_e is the ending age of the age group, and r is the rate observed for this age group.

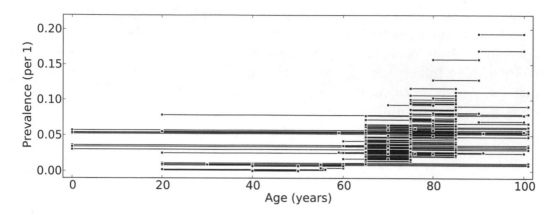

Figure 5.2. The systematic review of the descriptive epidemiology of atrial fibrillation included 155 observations of disease prevalence for the US. The prevalence level and age group of each observation are shown as a horizontal bar, with the position of the bar along the y-axis representing the prevalence level and the endpoints along the x-axis representing the start and end of the age group. The data show heterogeneity by age that is typical for these systematic review results and that clearly increases with age.

A brief word about a_e is in order here. Often in the epidemiological literature, the ending ages are described in a unit-dependent fashion, for example, age group 10–14. This is intended to mean from the first day of age 10 to the last day of age 14. However, this notation can be a hindrance when dealing with age resolution finer than 1 year, a situation that comes up when studying neonatal conditions. For this reason, I prefer the approach that takes the end age of the interval to be the first age when an individual is no longer part of the group. In the case above, I would say $a_e = 15$.

With a firm understanding of the sort of overlapping age-group data that arise in systematic review, I now turn to developing and analyzing a series of models for the meta-analysis of the data. I will consider five: the midpoint model, the disaggregation model, the midpoint-with-covariate model, the age-standardizing model, and the age-integrating model. The age-standardizing model is the balance of theoretical foundations, practical implementability, and empirical success that is used in the second half of this book.

5.2 Midpoint model

The simplest approach to modeling data with heterogeneous age intervals is to apply each rate measurement to the midpoint of the age group it measures. This is trivial operationally, but it is also theoretically justified through a "trapezoidal rule" integration.

In practice, this approach is quite accurate for modeling a disease rate that changes slowly as a function of age. However, it becomes inaccurate when modeling rates that change more rapidly. The typical setting in applications in the second half of this book will include both a few studies that focus on age patterns and hence have narrow age groups and also many studies that focus on other aspects of disease epidemiology. Thus, when considering how these models are inaccurate, the relevant setting is where there are a few small age-group studies and many large age-group studies.

Mathematically, the formulation is as follows: let $h(a)$ be a process model for the age-specific function (e.g., a spline model from Chapter 3 or the age-specific prevalence function derived from the solution to the system of differential equations from Section 7.2), and let $\mathbf{p}(r, n \mid \mu, \rho)$ be a data model for the observed level (e.g., the probability density function for the negative-binomial rate model from Chapter 2). Then the likelihood of an observation of rate r_i with effective sample size n_i for age group (a_{si}, a_{ei}) is simply $\mathbf{p}\left(r_i, n_i \mid h\left(\frac{a_{si}+a_{ei}}{2}\right), \rho\right)$. Equivalently, in "blackboard notation," using $\mathcal{D}(\mu, \rho; n_i)$ to denote the rate model distribution, I can write

$$r_i \sim \mathcal{D}\left(h(a_i), \rho; n_i\right),$$
$$a_i = \frac{a_{si} + a_{ei}}{2}.$$

This formulation will be convenient for comparison with the other models of age groups to come.

To understand how accurately age-group models like the midpoint model can estimate, I used simulation. The precise details are deferred until Section 5.6, but since this simulation is also used for the figures that follow, I will describe it briefly here. First, I selected an age-specific hazard function as truth. Then I generated noisy measurements from a mixture of regularly spaced 10-year age groups and uniformly random age groups. For each measurement, I chose a random population structure and integrated the true age-specific hazard to find the true rate for the age group. Then I sampled from a negative-binomial distribution with this true rate as the mean and a fixed overdispersion parameter to obtain noisy data, which I used in the age-group model. Since truth is known in this simulation, I can compare the model estimates to the truth graphically as well as quantitatively.

Figure 5.3 compares the estimate produced by the midpoint model to truth through simulation using two different age-specific hazard functions as truth. When the age-specific hazard varies little as a function of age, as shown in panel (a), the estimated hazard function is quite accurate. But when the age-specific hazard function varies substantially, as shown in panel (b), the estimate is biased.

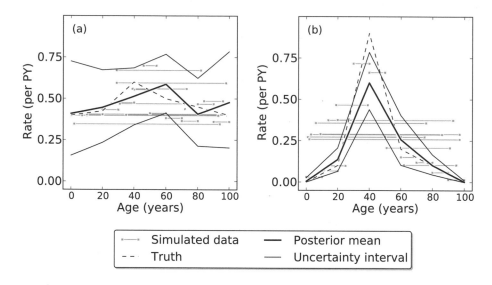

Figure 5.3. The midpoint model, a conceptually simple approach to dealing with data with heterogeneous age groups, simply attributes the observation to the midpoint of the age group. Panel (a) shows the model applied to an age-specific hazard function that does not vary a great deal across ages; the midpoint model is an accurate fit. Panel (b) shows the model applied to a more variable age-specific hazard function; the midpoint model overcompresses the estimates.

5.3 Disaggregation model

An alternative to the midpoint model that seems appealing but has some downsides is what I call *disaggregation*. To understand the disaggregation approach, imagine the simple reanalysis that I could do if microdata were available (as described at the beginning of this chapter). If I had access to the individual measurements that went into the calculation of the disease rate found in systematic review, I could do a reanalysis with any age grouping I wished. I could calculate rates for single-year age groups and be sure that the age pattern does not change substantially during the grouping.

The microdata from rates found in systematic review are rarely available, however. The disaggregation approach is a simple attempt to impute what the rates for the desired age grouping would be *if* the microdata were available. This requires taking into account the increased variation that would be found if a study of the same size was reported for finer age groups.

Without any additional information, rate data reporting a level of r for a population with effective sample size n for age group (a_s, a_e), that is,

$$X = (r, n, a_s, a_e)$$

can be disaggregated into $A = a_e - a_s$ rows of data, $X_1, X_2, \ldots, X_A$, with

$$X_a = \left(r, \frac{n}{a_e - a_s}, a, a + 1 \right), \text{ for } a = 1, 2, \ldots, A.$$

Disaggregation can be interpreted as a data-preprocessing step, and these disaggregated data can be fed into the midpoint model from the previous section to produce a comprehensive estimate of the rate as a function of age. However, this model has some unintended negative features when large age intervals are disaggregated. Because it ignores the correlation of disease levels with age, it tends to overcompress age patterns at young and old ages, as shown with simulated data in Figure 5.4.

5.4 Midpoint model with group width covariate

An alternative method, which I consider more "statistical" in its approach, is to add the width of the age group as a covariate into the midpoint model.

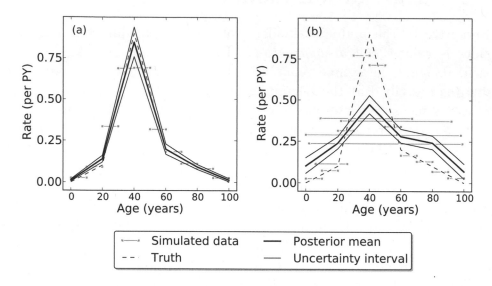

Figure 5.4. The disaggregation approach to two simulated datasets. In (a) the age groups are sufficiently fine-grained and homogeneous, and disaggregation is a successful approach. But in (b) with even slight heterogeneity, the model estimates are overcompressed.

This model takes the form

$$r_i \sim \mathcal{D}\left(\mu_i, \rho; n_i\right),$$
$$\mu_i = h\left(\frac{a_{si} + a_{ei}}{2}\right) + \theta(a_e - a_s).$$

This addresses the shortcomings of the disaggregation approach *indirectly*, and the indirect nature has positives and negatives. This method does not explicitly connect the large age interval to the small age interval but instead allows the data to inform the relationship. On the other hand, it posits that the data-driven relationship between the rates for studies with the same midpoint but different age groups is a linear relationship. In contrast, the mathematical model developed at the beginning of this chapter is nonlinear in a specific and mechanistically known way. Figure 5.5 shows the results of applying the midpoint-covariate model to simulated data.

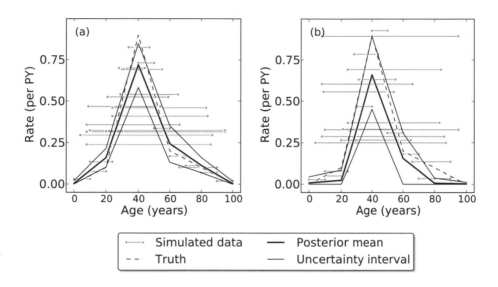

Figure 5.5. The midpoint-covariate model applied to two simulated datasets, where truth is known. Although this approach is appealing theoretically, the added flexibility of the covariate model does not add much value in the simulation study.

5.5   Age-standardizing and age-integrating models

An even more complicated approach, both conceptually and computationally, is to average across the age interval explicitly in the statistical model:

$$r_i \sim \mathcal{D}\left(\mu_i, \rho; n_i\right),$$
$$\mu_i = \int_{a=a_{s_i}}^{a_{e_i}} h(a)\mathbf{d}w_i(a),$$

where the integration $\mathbf{d}w_i$ is weighted according to population structure.

This has the theoretical appeal of matching the generative model above but the drawback of being slower computationally and less stable numerically. It also has a major piece left unspecified: the selection of the age weights for the integration. There are two sensible approaches to age-weight selection, which I call the *age-standardizing model* and the *age-integrating model*. The age-standardizing model uses a common age-specific weight function $\mathbf{d}w_i(a) = \mathbf{d}w(a)$ for all studies, while the age-integrating model uses the best estimate available of the age pattern of the study population in each observation. The age-standardizing model is faster, due to a computational optimization only possible when the $\mathbf{d}w_i$ are the same for all i, but the age-integrating model is appealing on theoretical grounds, because it can use more information. However, it is not certain that using this information will make the end results any more accurate, because the age pattern of the study population is not always known with great certainty, and then it is necessary to assume that it matches the national age pattern for the country-years where the study was conducted. In the case of remission and mortality studies it is even more complicated to estimate the study population age pattern, since it is *not* the same as the national population age pattern but modulated by the age pattern of disease prevalence. Figure 5.6 shows the results of the age-standardizing model on simulated data.

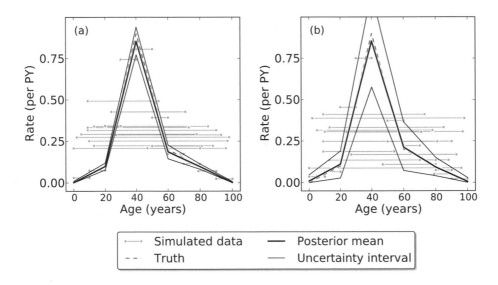

Figure 5.6. The age-standardizing model applied to simulated data with a known age-specific rate function as truth. The results in panel (a) show that the model recovers the true age pattern quite precisely. Panel (b) shows that the results are still accurate when the data-generation procedure is even more noisy.

5.6 Model comparison

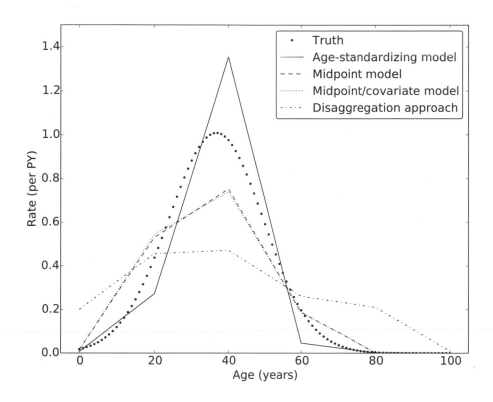

Figure 5.7. A comparison of four models for heterogeneous age groups shows that the age-standardizing model comes closest to recovering the truth. This corresponds to the results of the simulation study presented in Table 5.1.

An appropriate comparison of these approaches is somewhat difficult to develop. One approach is through simulation, where a dataset is simulated from known truth (Figure 5.7). This allows the estimates to be compared to "true" values, but this risks inappropriate model selection due to inaccurately choosing the distribution of the simulated data. Another approach is cross-validation, where data from systematic review are split into mutually exclusive *training* and *test* sets, and the model is fitted to the training set and used to predict the values in the test set. Naively holding out 25% of the data does not address the exact topic of interest, however, since it determines which model predicts rates of all age groups, and I am really only interested in predicting the age groups with small widths accurately. It would be preferable to hold out only data with small-width age groups from large representative subpopulations. Unfortunately, there are rarely enough data to do this, especially in all the settings that come up in disease modeling.

I have taken a pragmatic approach, evaluating by means of the natural simulation described below. Future work, based on more sophisticated simulation scenarios or based on carefully designed holdout cross-validation, is necessary to further understand the trade-offs between these alternative methods.

The data simulation procedure I used is the following:

- Choose age intervals for 30 rows of data; for $i = 1, \ldots, 10$, $(a_{si}, a_{ei}) = (10(i-1), 10i)$, and for the remaining 20 intervals, choose the age interval width uniformly at random from $[1, 100]$ and choose the midpoint of the age interval uniformly at random from ages compatible with this age range.

- Choose the effective sample size n_i for each row uniformly at random from $[10^2, 10^4]$.

- Choose an age-specific population structure for each row of data, with the form $w_i(a) = e^{\beta_i a}$, where β_i is drawn from a normal distribution with mean 0 and standard deviation $\frac{1}{10}$.

- Calculate the true rate value for each age interval,

$$r_i^{\text{true}} = \sum_{a=a_{si}}^{a_{ei}} \mu_{\text{true}}(a) w_i(a),$$

where

$$\mu_{\text{true}}(a) = \exp\left\{\frac{3(a-35)^2}{1000} + \frac{a-35}{100}\right\}.$$

- Choose an observed rate value, based on a negative binomial distribution: $r_i n_i \sim \text{NegativeBinomial}(r_i^{\text{true}}, \delta_{\text{true}})$, where $\delta_{\text{true}} = 5$.

Table 5.1 shows the median results of fitting these simulated data for a variety of models. The age-standardizing model is superior in all metrics of fit quality.

Table 5.1. Median results for 100 replicates of the simulation study comparing age-specific rate estimates from five models of age-grouped data.

Model	Bias (pp)	MAE (pp)	PC (%)	Time (s)
Midpoint	3	6	60	32
Disaggregation	−1	22	5	40
Midpoint-covariate	4	6	72	37
Age-standardizing	0	3	75	34
Age-integrating	0	3	70	35

Note: Bias is the mean of truth minus predicted measured in percentage points (pp), median absolute error (MAE) is the median of absolute difference between truth and predicted, probability of coverage (PC) is the fraction of truth falling within 95% uncertainty interval of prediction, and time is the computation time.

5.7 Summary and future work

This chapter has developed and compared several alternative approaches to dealing with heterogeneous age groups in systematic review data. Although the age-standardizing model has been preferred on theoretical grounds and simulation study, future work comparing the performance of these approaches at out-of-sample prediction is necessary to confirm this choice. Additional approaches to age group heterogeneity based on alternative statistical or machine learning methods may also be worthwhile.

Chapter 6

Covariate modeling

Abraham D. Flaxman

Covariate modeling is a method to explain the variation in noisy data in terms of demographic, epidemiological, and study-specific variables. The term "covariate" emerged in the 1940s, and one of its first appearances is in the proceedings of a meeting of the Royal Statistical Society,[63] describing an approach to measuring agricultural output indirectly. By making a number of measurements of weights of the same jade plant immediately after harvest and again after the plant dried, P.C. Mahalanobis was able to derive a relationship between the easier to measure, but less relevant, weight immediately after harvesting and the more important, but less available, weight when the goods were ready for market. This "method of covariates" is the same in spirit of the covariate modeling we still use today. However, we are often faced with even less flexibility about what to measure. The meaning of the term covariate will become clearer through its use over the course of this chapter.

Using covariates in global disease burden estimation is challenging because there is often no particularly explanatory variable available. To understand this, the jade plant example where the term first emerged may be instructive. Conceptually, it should be possible to predict the dry weight of plants very precisely without measuring it directly after drying. If the farmer knows the weight when harvested, the water content of the plant, the humidity over the growing season, and the storage conditions after harvest, it is plausible that chemistry and physics can combine all of this information and make a second weighing unnecessary. However, when not all of this information is available, it is still possible to make a rougher estimate, and the theory of statistics is very good at doing so and even quantifying how rough the estimate will be. In many applications during the GBD 2010 study, there was not even a covariate as related as the harvest weight, and we considered the utility of indirectly associated predictors like gross domestic product per capita or average rainfall. In many applications, covariates were used quite analogously to the harvest weight of the plants as well, however.

In my metaregression model of disease in populations, covariate modeling has two distinct goals. One is to explain the bias and variation of the noisy measurements of epidemiological rates. For example, covariates can be used as a mechanism for data-driven "cross-walks" to convert between alternative diagnostic methods that have different sensitivities, and covariates can also be used to objectively down-weight data that come from a noisier source, such as nonrepresentative subpopulations when they are not systematically biased above or below the mean. In a Bayesian context, these covariates serve to make the studies more exchangeable.

The other goal in covariate modeling is to increase the accuracy of out-of-sample predictions. This is accomplished by modeling the relationships between the disease parameters of interest and the explanatory covariates. The modeled relationships are then used to extrapolate predictions for the disease parameters to geographic regions where covariate data are available but where no or few direct measurements have been made.

In covariate modeling, a distinction is often made between "fixed effects" and "random effects." Bayesian approaches, such as hierarchical modeling, blur this distinction. To make the nomenclature more complicated, different methodological traditions of covariate modeling have opposite concepts of what is fixed and what is random in effects.

For this metaregression framework, I have used fixed and random effects in different ways, which makes them easy to keep separated. While I have used fixed effects for covariates that vary by study or by country-year, I have used random effects to model only indicator covariates for geographic units.

Sometimes I have constrained the random effects to sum to zero at each level of a geographic hierarchy, which is an extension of the traditional meaning of random effects in linear regression, where the population mean of a random effect is zero. In other models, it is sufficient to use a prior with mean zero independently for each random effect, as is the common approach in Bayesian modeling. In either case, my random effects always have a hyperparameter for the dispersion, which allows the model to infer how dispersed the random effects are between geographic regions and hence to quantify the uncertainty in the geographic regions for which no data are available.

The fixed effects thus model variation between measurements that can be explained, while the random effects model true variation between measurements for which we have no explanatory covariates. Distinct from both of these is the model for sampling and nonsampling variation in the measurements, which is implicit in the rate models developed in Chapter 2. In the case of a negative binomial rate model with random effects, for example, the model must distinguish between true variation from country to country and nonsampling variation. This is quite a challenge when limited data are available.

I will develop all these concepts in the following sections of this chapter.

6.1 Cross-walk fixed effects to explain bias

The first use of covariate modeling that we will investigate is the cross-walk, where study-specific fixed effects are used to combine measurements of different but multiplicatively related quantities. A prototypical example comes from myocardial infarction (MI) incidence, where a variety of diagnostic tests are available. Different studies of MI incidence use different diagnostic criteria for case ascertainment. The newer class of tests, which are based on measuring levels of the blood protein troponin, are more sensitive than earlier methods, and this leads to variation in data with a clear explanation. Figure 6.1 shows simulated data with a covariate that has an effect like a troponin-based test might, raising the number of observed cases by 30%. By including an indicator variable as a covariate in each row of data, $x_i = 1$ if row i comes from a study that used a troponin test, and $x_i = 0$ otherwise, I can fit a model that includes a parameter to cross-walk between studies using these two different case ascertainment criteria.

This same approach can be applied to data on mental disorders gathered with different recall periods, an application that arises frequently in the meta-analysis of psychological disorders. For example, in measuring the population prevalence of bipolar disorder, many studies ask about symptoms in the past month, while many others ask about the past year. Figure 6.2 shows the data collected in systematic review for bipolar disorder, where past-year prevalence is higher than past-month prevalence because of the episodic nature of the condition.

In general, let the data collected in systematic review be denoted by tuples (a_i, n_i, r_i, X_i), where a_i is the age group, n_i is the effective sample size, r_i is

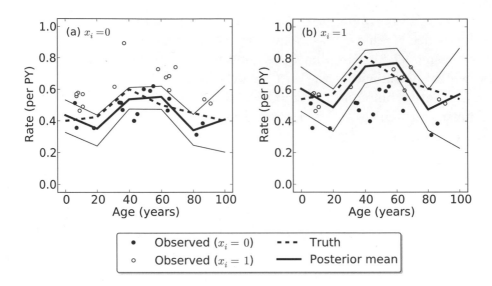

Figure 6.1. Simulated dataset where different measurement techniques yield systematically different values. The data with $x_i = 1$ are on average 30% higher than data with $x_i = 0$, and the covariate model recovers this difference accurately, with sufficient data. Panels (a) and (b) show the same data. (a) shows the true and predicted values for $x_i = 0$ and (b) shows the true and predicted values for $x_i = 1$.

the observed rate value, and X_i is a vector of covariate values. Then, using $\mathcal{D}(\pi, \rho; n_i)$ to denote the rate model (with $\mathcal{D}$ to denote a general distribution for the data likelihood), the fixed-effects covariate model is

$$r_i \sim \mathcal{D}\left(\mu_i, \delta; n_i\right),$$
$$\mu_i = h(a_i)e^{\beta X_i}$$

The parameter β represents the effect coefficients for the fixed effects, and it can help the stability of the computational algorithms to put a diffuse prior on β, such as

$$\beta_j \sim \text{Normal}\left(0, \sigma_j^2\right) \text{ for } j = 1, \ldots, J.$$

Of course, if experts have beliefs about the sign or magnitude of the effect coefficient, this can be included as a more informative prior.

Two subtle choices are worth additional investigation in fixed-effects modeling: normalization and reference values. Both of these choices are known to

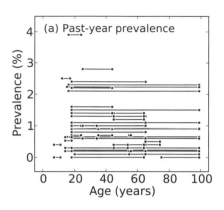 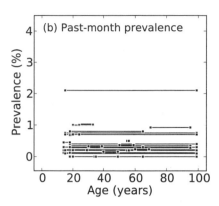

Figure 6.2. Data on bipolar disorder collected in systematic review. Some studies measured past-year prevalence, while others measured past-month prevalence. Because of the episodic nature of the condition, past-month prevalence is 30%–40% lower than past-year prevalence.

influence the performance of computational algorithms.[37] For example, non-normalized covariates can produce nonconvergence in hill-climbing algorithms that work fine with normalized covariates. But because of the Bayesian priors and especially because of the consistency from the compartmental model, the choices are particularly important in this setting. When the covariates have been normalized to have mean zero and standard deviation 1, taking $\sigma_j = 1$ in the diffuse prior above seems to work well in practice.

The term *reference value* is borrowed from fixed-effects modeling of categorical variables, where so-called dummy variables (0/1 indicators) are introduced for all but one category. When all the dummy covariates are set to zero, the model produces predictions for the reference category. In the formulation above, the analogous notion occurs when $X_i = (0, 0, \ldots, 0)$. Then the expression for μ_i simplifies to

$$\mu_i = h(a_i)e^{\beta \mathbf{0}} = h(a_i).$$

It is this h that is used as the age-specific rate function in the compartmental model (as developed in Chapter 7), so the consistency between incidence, prevalence, remission, and mortality is enforced at the reference values.

Because the reference values are consistent, they must be chosen with care. For example, in the case of MI above, where some studies used troponin-based diagnostics and some did not, the reference value should be *with* troponin tests, because this is considered to be more accurate.

A concrete example using the bipolar disorder data can make this clearer. Chapter 14 provides another example, while Chapter 19 develops the consistent model for bipolar disorder in detail, which is used here in two variations: when the past-year prevalence is used as the reference value, and when the past-month prevalence is used as the reference value. This changes the predicted prevalence, of course, but it also changes the predicted incidence (for which few data are available). Figure 6.3 shows how the alternative reference values change the incidence estimate in this case.

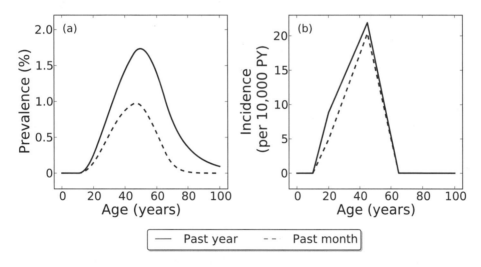

Figure 6.3. The reference value for the past-year/past-month prevalence covariate has a substantial effect on incidence estimates. Because consistency is enforced at the reference value level, choosing reference values is an important modeling decision.

Normalization is also important, although it does not affect consistency. It is important for stability of numerical algorithms and also because the prior on the effect coefficient must be matched to the scale of the covariate. Normalizing continuous covariates to have variance 1, for example, means that the prior of $\beta \sim \text{Normal}(0, 1^2)$ is diffuse. If a continuous covariate had variance 0.0001, the same prior on β would be very informative.

6.2 Predictive fixed effects to improve out-of-sample estimation

In addition to study-level covariates, like the cross-walks in the previous section, covariate modeling can be used at the areal level to use relationships measured in-sample to improve estimation of true regional variation out-of-sample. Mathematically, the setting is identical, where an areal-level covariate matrix X_i' holds the value of the covariates, and an effect coefficient parameter β' controls the prediction, multiplying h by $e^{\beta' X_i'}$. Conceptually, this deserves separate treatment, however, because the use and the results of areal-level covariate modeling are quite different.

The benefit of using fixed effects to predict out-of-sample is clear when modeling an often fatal condition, like decompensated cirrhosis. Incidence of this disease is available from registries for some regions, but population-level mortality caused by the condition has been modeled in detail for all countries.[19] By using the log of the age-standardized mortality rate as a covariate in the incidence model, it is possible to borrow strength from the mortality estimates to inform the incidence estimates. Chapter 15 explores this specific example in more detail.

This approach can also be helpful for covariates that are not as direct, for example, using gross domestic product as an explanatory covariate for estimating the prevalence of eating disorders, using estimates of age-standardized hepatitis C virus prevalence as an explanatory covariate for estimating prevalence of cirrhosis, or using an indicator for violent conflict as an explanatory covariate for estimating the prevalence of depression and anxiety disorder.

However, to use areal-level covariates in this way requires having a time series with areal-level data for each area and year of study included in the analysis. These data may be sparse and noisy as well, and often require imputation for missing areal or year values.

6.3 Fixed effects to explain variance

Fixed-effects modeling in the previous sections has focused on improving predictions of the mean of observed data. It is also possible to use fixed-effects modeling to explain the different levels of variation in different sources of data, which is the topic of this section.

To introduce this idea by way of example, consider the results of a systematic review for hepatitis C virus seroprevalence. This literature search excluded studies in subpopulations known to have systematic bias, such as studies of prevalence in intravenous drug users or paid blood donors. But it did collect measurements from studies in subpopulations that were *not* known to be systematically biased, for example, studies that used voluntary blood donors as the sample frame. This is clearly not the whole population, but as it is not known to be a biased sample, I would like to include it if possible. This is where using a fixed effect to explain variation is appropriate. The systematic review assigned a bias indicator $Z_i = 1$ to observations corresponding to the voluntary blood donors, as well as to observations from other studies of nonrepresentative subpopulations, such as mothers visiting antenatal clinics. Observations from studies of the general population received bias indicator $Z_i = 0$. Then I was able to introduce a fixed-effect coefficient analogous to that discussed in the previous sections, but modifying the overdispersion term of the rate model instead of the mean.

This procedure resulted in the following formulation:

$$r_i \sim \mathcal{D}\left(\mu_i, \delta_i; n_i\right),$$
$$\mu_i = h(a_i)e^{\beta X_i},$$
$$\delta_i = e^{\eta + \zeta Z_i}.$$

6.4 Random effects for spatial variation

Another important use of covariates is in handling nonsampling variation that *cannot* be explained. As I have mentioned repeatedly, the descriptive epidemiological data available are often very noisy. Usually only a small part of this "noise" can be explained with covariates like those from the preceding section. And while the additional variation has no simple explanation in terms of differing diagnostic criteria or the like, there is structure in the variation. Countries in the North Africa and Middle East region have rates more similar to each other than to countries in the high-income North America region. And the high-income North America region as a whole is more similar to the Western Europe region than to the South Asia region. Capturing this spatial similarity when it exists is the goal in my random-effects modeling.

I will develop this approach to random-effects modeling by beginning with something very similar to the fixed-effects model. The random effects come, in part, through the use of an additional parameter in the model and additional factors in the prior, either modeling the dispersion of the effects as a parameter itself to be fitted from the data or going further to model the joint distribution of spatially neighboring effects to have group means equal to 0. For notation, let U_i be a vector of random-effects covariates. This U_i is a *design matrix* analogous to the fixed-effect covariate vector X_i above, but with 0/1 values corresponding to the place in the spatial hierarchy to which observation i refers.

In the GBD 2010 study, the spatial hierarchy is countries nested in regions nested in superregions, but in national or subnational analyses, the hierarchy will be different. This can be generically formulated using graph theory, but the precise graph-theoretic details are not necessary for this exposition.

Analogously to the fixed-effects model above, the random effects apply a multiplicative shift to the age-specific rate function:

$$r_i \sim \mathcal{D}\left(\mu_i, \delta_i; n_i\right),$$
$$\mu_i = h(a_i)e^{\alpha U_i}.$$

The first difference between the fixed effects and random effects is in the priors on the effect coefficients. Instead of a diffuse prior as used above for the fixed effects, the prior on α is itself part of the model, parametrized as

$$\alpha_j \sim \text{Normal}\left(0, \sigma_{\ell(j)}^2\right),$$

where $\ell(j)$ is the level in the hierarchy of area j, and σ_ℓ is also a model parameter, representing the standard deviation of the area-to-area variation between areas at level ℓ in the hierarchy. To fit this model with Bayesian methods, we also need a prior on σ_ℓ (a hyperprior), and this often has to be somewhat informative. The truncated normal distribution

$$\sigma_\ell \sim \text{Normal}_{[0.05,5]}\left(0.05, 0.03^2\right),$$

is often an appropriate choice. It says that between-area variation with standard deviation of less than 5% is impossible and more than 15% is rare.

A second difference between the fixed effects and random effects that can help with MCMC convergence is the following modification to the joint prior distribution of (α_j): for every group of areas nested within a common area in the spatial hierarchy (for example, all countries in the same region), I can constrain the random effects for the group to have mean 0. Using $A_1, \ldots, A_J$

to denote all groups of areal regions nested in a common super-area, this constraint can be formalized mathematically as

$$\sum_{a \in A_j} \alpha_a = 0, \text{ for } A_1, A_2, \ldots, A_J$$

The group mean centering prior has important implications in consistent models, because as described above (and shown in Figure 6.3), consistency is enforced at the reference level, which for random effects is $U_i = \mathbf{0}$. The group mean centering constraint has the benefit of reducing the number of dimensions in the parameter space, which is why it helps with MCMC convergence.

6.5   Covariates and consistency

One of the most challenging theoretical issues in covariate modeling for integrative systems modeling is the interplay between the predictive covariates and the intercompartmental consistency. The exposition of this challenging concept is further complicated because the compartmental model to which the intercompartmental consistency applies has not yet been developed in detail (it appears in Chapter 7). However, it seems best for reference purposes to include this material here, and first-time readers should proceed knowing that it will be easier the second time around.

A simple example of the problem arises in a model of congenital abnormalities, where there is birth prevalence, prevalence at older ages, and mortality risk, but there is no incidence or remission after birth. If covariates are used to shift predictions for the level of $h_{p \cdot f}$ as well as the level of h_p and the level of h_f, then consistency would require that $\beta_i^{h_{p \cdot f}} = \beta_i^{h_p} + \beta_i^{h_f}$.

This complication becomes even more pronounced in a model with nonzero incidence and remission. In the general case, it is not even clear that nonzero covariate effects exist that respect consistency.

To circumvent this challenge, I have used a multistage approach to fitting the model (see Section 8.7), and at each stage of the process, there is a specific level of the hierarchical model where I have enforced the consistency conditions of the system dynamics model. All predictions from this stage apply only to this area and areas grouped within it in the spatial hierarchy. For the subareas, however, the predictions are not consistent. They are expected to be close to consistent, a hypothesis that must be investigated empirically on a case-by-case basis.

How does this work? Recall the covariate model formulation for predicting the rate for a given geographic area, sex, and year (g, s, y):

$$\boldsymbol{\pi}_{g,s,y}(a) = h(a)e^{\alpha U_{g,s,y} + \beta X_{g,s,y}}.$$

For the top level of the spatial hierarchy (also called the *reference node* and corresponding to geographic area, sex, and year, (g_r, s_r, y_r)), I simply apply a linear shift to each covariate in X and U so that $X_{g_r,s_r,y_r} = \mathbf{0}$ and $U_{g_r,s_r,y_r} = \mathbf{0}$. This simplifies to

$$\boldsymbol{\pi}_{g_r,s_r,y_r}(a) = h(a),$$

and for any system of differential equations for which $\{h_t(a), t = [T]\}$ are solutions, the predicted values for the age, sex, and year at the root of the hierarchy are also solutions.

An important direction for future work is to go beyond the multistage approach. This will probably require innovation in algorithms, because fitting multiple consistent models simultaneously is currently impractical.

6.6   Summary and future work

This chapter described the multiple ways covariates have been used in descriptive epidemiological metaregression: to explain bias, to improve the accuracy of out-of-sample prediction, to explain variance, and to measure unexplained variation. These different applications are all similar mathematically, but there is much subtlety in how each influences the model estimates.

In future work, it will be important to develop covariates that themselves include uncertainty, since many predictive covariates are themselves estimates. Similarly, methods that allow covariates with missing values will be useful in future modeling efforts. The covariate modeling developed in the Cause of Death portion of the Global Burden of Disease 2010 study benefited greatly from ensemble modeling methods,[19] an additional approach that could be tried here as well.

Chapter 7

Prevalence estimates from other data types

Abraham D. Flaxman

Often the results of a systematic review contain measurements of disease parameters that cannot be combined directly. The example on Parkinson's disease in the Introduction included data on disease prevalence and incidence, and not enough of either. It would be quite unfortunate if we had to pick just one at a time to look at. Fortunately, this is not the case. Disease incidence, prevalence, remission, and mortality are intimately linked, and in this chapter I will develop a method to bring these diverse data together in a single model. This provides estimates that are informed by all available data and helps to identify when different types of measurements produce information that is consistent and when they are inconsistent.

To inform age-specific estimates of prevalence with data on other epidemiological parameters (such as incidence, remission, and mortality), this chapter introduces the framework that I call *integrative systems modeling* (ISM). ISM combines a mechanistic model of process with a statistical model of data. The foundations of ISM are best articulated in terms of *system dynamics modeling*, a discipline that originated in the fields of operations research and industrial engineering.[64,65,66,67] This type of compartmental modeling is similar to infectious disease modeling[68,69,70,71,72] and pharmacokinetic/pharmacodynamic (PK/PD) modeling.[73,74,75,76,77,78]

System dynamics modeling is a method to model the behavior of complex systems in terms of stocks, flows, and feedback loops. In short, *stock variables* quantify the amount of some material, mass, or population in a compartment at a particular moment in time, while *flow variables* quantify the rate of material moving into, out of, or between compartments. The scope of applications for system dynamics is enormous, and once you start thinking of systems in this way, it may seem that everything can be modeled as stocks and flows. This method has been applied to the study of complex systems in economics, politics, environmental science, and a diverse array of other fields.[67,77,79,80]

Traditionally, there is a delineation between system dynamics modeling and statistical modeling: system dynamics aims to develop a *model of process*, while statistical approaches focus on developing a *model of data*. Models of process attempt to explicitly represent the mechanisms behind some system behavior (deterministically or stochastically), while models of data often explicitly avoid requiring such a theory. The advantage of using the system dynamics approach is that it can incorporate structural assumptions about the system. However, in many applications, the system dynamics model of process is not connected to data at all. On the other hand, in many statistical approaches, the domain-specific dynamics of the system under study are not incorporated in the model explicitly, and this exclusion may be intentional, to allow the data to speak for themselves. In the case of sparse and noisy data, data models could benefit from additional structure. ISM is a framework to bring together a model of process and a model of data for mutual benefit: the model of data is used to estimate the parameters for the model of process.

7.1   A motivating example: population dynamics

An example will help to make these concepts more concrete. We begin with the simplest of compartmental models, a single compartment with inflow, outflow, and no feedback, shown schematically in Figure 7.1.

Schematic diagrams of stock-and-flow models such as Figure 7.1 are useful in understanding and communicating the structure of a model of process, but the full description is best represented in the form of a system of difference equations or differential equations that specify precisely the relationship between the stocks and flows. The following differential equation fully specifies the one-compartment model:

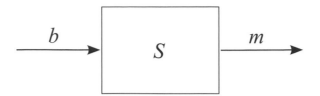

Figure 7.1. A single-compartment model with inflow b and outflow m is one of the simplest examples of a compartmental model. Despite its simplicity, it is a useful model of population dynamics. In this application, b represents births, m represents mortality, while S represents the "stock" of population.

$$\frac{dS}{dt} = b - m,$$
$$b = h_b S,$$
$$m = h_m S.$$

In this equation, the stock S changes continuously, increasing with birth hazard h_b and decreasing with mortality hazard h_m. When h_b and h_m are constants with respect to time, this differential equation has a closed-form solution: $S = S_0 e^{(h_b - h_m)t}$. When h_b and h_m are not constant with respect to time, the model does not necessarily have a closed-form solution, and many more time trends are possible for S. Panel (a) of Figure 7.2 shows the time trend of S when h_b and h_m are constant; panel (b) shows the time trend when they are changing.

The next section focuses on the specific application that is crucial to model-based metaregression: the system dynamics of a disease moving through a population, with flows that vary as a function of age.

7.2 System dynamics model of disease in a population

The key to combining data of different types is a two-compartment system dynamics model of process. The compartments contain the population susceptible to the disease (stock S, for "susceptible") and the population with the condition (stock C, for "condition"). The population moves between these

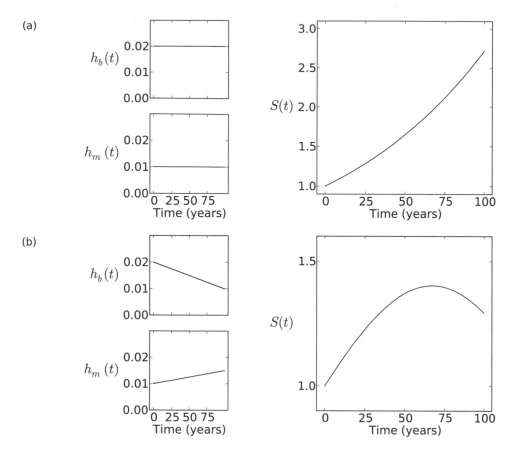

Figure 7.2. Stock and flow in a one-compartment model as a function of time. Panel (a) shows the exponentially growing stock when inflow and outflow hazards are constant with respect to time, and the inflow exceeds the outflow. Panel (b) shows the nonmonotonic change in stock with respect to time in a system where the inflow hazard is decreasing as a function of time and the outflow hazard is increasing.

compartments following the arrows shown in Figure 7.3, transitioning from S to C with incidence hazard h_i, and from C back to S with remission hazard h_r. The susceptible population flows out of the system with background mortality hazard h_m, and the with-condition population flows out of the system with with-condition mortality hazard $h_{m_{\text{with}}} = h_m + h_f$. Here h_f represents the "excess mortality hazard" for individuals with the condition over individuals without the condition.[9]

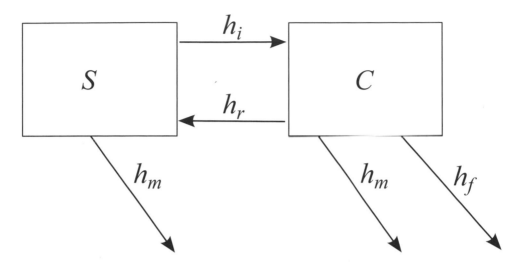

Figure 7.3. The two-compartment model of process for disease in a population, which allows prevalence estimates to be informed by other types of data. Compartment S contains the population susceptible to the disease, and compartment C contains the population with the condition. Individuals move from S to C with incidence hazard h_i, and from C to S with remission hazard h_r. The susceptible population flows out of the system with without-condition mortality hazard h_m, and the with-condition population flows out of the system with with-condition mortality hazard $h_m + h_f$, where h_f is the excess mortality hazard and represents quantitatively the increase in mortality for individuals with the condition.

This "model of process" looks deceptively simple, and compared to the complex systems often developed in infectious disease modeling it *is* quite simple. However, it is more flexible than it appears at first glance. All the parameters of the model are functions of age and time, which permits enough flexibility to match well the myriad of available data about the descriptive epidemiology of disease. I will connect this model of process to data using the age-standardizing mixed-effects spline models from the previous chapters, and together they will provide the integrative systems model for metaregression that incorporates data on parameters other than prevalence into a prevalence estimate.

As mentioned in the previous section, a schematic depiction of a compartmental model, such as Figure 7.3, is not a complete description of the system dynamics. To specify them completely requires a system of differential equations that correspond to the stocks and flows above and that more precisely represent their relationship as a function of time and age, using variable τ to capture the fact that cohorts age together as time progresses:

$$\frac{d}{d\tau}S(a+\tau, t+\tau) = -(h_i + h_m)S + h_r C,$$

$$\frac{d}{d\tau}C(a+\tau, t+\tau) = h_i S - (h_r + h_m + h_f)C.$$

The notation $S, C, h_i, h_r, h_m,$ and h_f denote the following functions of age and time:

$S = S(a, t) =$ stock of "susceptibles,"

$C = C(a, t) =$ stock of "with condition,"

$h_i = h_i(a, t) =$ incidence hazard for susceptibles (S),

$h_r = h_r(a, t) =$ remission hazard for individuals with the condition (C),

$h_m = h_m(a, t) =$ (without-condition) mortality hazard for susceptibles (S),

$h_f = h_f(a, t) =$ excess mortality hazard for individuals with the condition (C).

Several quantities derived from these stocks and flows will also come up repeatedly in the following discussion, so I collect those here as well:

$p = p(a, t) = C/(S + C) =$ prevalence of condition,

$h_{m_{\text{all}}} = h_{m_{\text{all}}}(a, t) =$ all-cause mortality hazard for all individuals,

$h_{m_{\text{with}}} = h_{m_{\text{with}}}(a, t) = h_m + h_f =$ with-condition mortality hazard (C),

$RR = RR(a, t) = (h_m + h_f)/(h_m) =$ relative risk of mortality (C vs S),

$SMR = SMR(a, t) = (h_m + h_f)/h_{m_{\text{all}}} =$ standardized mortality ratio (C vs all),

$h_{p \cdot f} = h_{p \cdot f}(a, t) = p \cdot h_f =$ population-level excess mortality hazard,

$X = X(a, t) =$ average duration of condition.

In general, all these quantities are functions of both age a and time t.

The tradition of system dynamics modeling would now consider sources of feedback in the system and other drivers of complex patterns. Even with two compartments, four rates, and no feedback, there is a wide range of possible patterns of disease, so if we added feedback to the model things would become quite complicated. However, in ISM we now take a different course. At this point, the model of process is sufficiently rich to consider what descriptive epidemiological data may be collected in systematic review, and how these data will relate to the stocks and flows in the model.

For some highly infectious diseases, for example, tuberculosis, cases identified in the health system are regularly reported to WHO. This yields data on disease incidence rates (which are not age-specific rates but crude incidence rates over all ages). The number of cases per year divided by the midyear population provides an approximate measurement of the incidence hazard h_i in Figure 7.3.

Often it is prevalence that is directly measured, for example, through a household or telephone survey. This sort of research provides measurements of the form "k out of n respondents tested positive for the condition" (or said that they had the condition). From this, we can obtain a measurement of the ratio of compartments in the stock-and-flow model above: that is, prevalence p is equal to $C/(S + C)$. Often this information will be stratified by age, sex, or both, and for many important diseases, the prevalence level will vary by orders of magnitude over the age range of the population.

Another sort of study that is sometimes available measures the relative risk of mortality (also known as the relative mortality ratio) of a disease, meaning the mortality rate in people with the disease and without the disease, and reports the ratio (sometime called the relative risk). This corresponds to a ratio of hazards in the model above, $RR = (h_m + h_f)/h_m$. Unfortunately, h_f is rarely measured directly, but the with-condition mortality hazard is sometimes reported instead of relative mortality risk, which can be represented as $h_{m_{\text{with}}} = h_m + h_f$.

The all-cause mortality for a population is a quantity that can be measured without need to investigate a specific disease, and therefore it is often known more precisely than the other quantities introduced so far. It can be calculated from vital registration or survey data as the number of deaths in a year divided by the midyear population, although more sophisticated approaches have been developed for cases where these data are not available. In the GBD 2010 study, all-cause mortality was estimated in a completely separate exercise and was available as an additional data input. These data are easier to collect than morbidity data, and there is a strong tradition of collection and analysis in the field of demography.[81]

All-cause mortality can also be derived from the model, as follows:

$$
\begin{aligned}
h_{m_{\text{all}}} &= (1 - p) \cdot h_m + p \cdot h_{m_{\text{with}}} \\
&= \frac{S}{S + C} h_m + \frac{C}{S + C} (h_m + h_f) \\
&= h_m + \frac{C}{S + C} h_f \\
&= h_m + p \cdot h_f.
\end{aligned}
$$

The quantity $h_{p \cdot f} = p \cdot h_f$ is what I am calling the population-level excess mortality hazard. It is important in its own right, because in some important cases, it is equal to the cause-specific mortality rate. For conditions that are unambiguously coded as the cause of death on death certificates, the population-level cause-specific mortality rate (i.e., the number of death certificates with this cause coded as the underlying cause of death divided by the person-years lived) is approximately equal to this population-level excess mortality rate. Even for conditions where the death certificates are not likely to be coded to this cause for all deaths (e.g., diabetes), the cause-specific mortality rate is a lower bound on $h_{p \cdot f}$, which can still provide useful information.

An important distinction between the hazards $h_{m_{\text{with}}}$ and $h_{p \cdot f}$ is the population to which they apply. The hazard $h_{m_{\text{with}}}$ applies *only* to the with-condition population, while $h_{p \cdot f}$ applies to the general population, including both those with and those without the condition. The hazard $h_{m_{\text{with}}}$ can be measured by following a cohort of individuals with the condition over time, while $h_{p \cdot f}$ can sometimes be measured by looking at deaths due to the condition in the general population.

Remission and duration studies, in which individuals with the disease are tracked over time to estimate how long the disease persists, provide yet another measurement that corresponds to parameters in this model (in the case of remission) or a quantity that can be derived from the model parameters (in the case of duration).

Representing average duration of the condition (i.e., the expected time an individual spends in compartment C before leaving) is a relatively involved calculation, included here for completeness:

$$
\text{duration}(a, t) = \int_{\tau=0}^{\infty} e^{-\left(h_r(a+\tau, t+\tau) + h_f(a+\tau, t+\tau) + h_m(a+\tau, t+\tau)\right)\tau} \mathbf{d}\tau.
$$

This integral can be simplified considerably for certain special cases. For example, if the remission hazard is constant as a function of age and time, and the mortality hazards h_m and h_f are small, then the duration simplifies to $\int_{\tau \geq 0} e^{-h_r \tau} \mathrm{d}\tau = \frac{1}{h_r}$. This justifies the approximation that remission rate is nearly equal to 1 over duration in acute conditions.

The data available for these parameters varies widely among the diseases that have been analyzed in GBD 2010. Some diseases have more data, while others have only prevalence or only incidence and not much of that. These gaps and the bridges between what we know and what we want to know will be explored in theory and practice in several later sections of this book.

With this detour through potentially available data in mind, it is now instructive to return to the more challenging elements of the compartmental model. Conceptually, it is excess mortality hazard h_f that has proven hardest to explain and to understand. It can be interpreted as the difference between the mortality rates in the cases and controls in a cohort study. For this measurement of h_f to be accurate, however, the study must avoid selection bias, which is quite a challenge in observational studies. Perhaps it would be clearer to focus on the with-condition mortality hazard, which can be measured directly in cohort study. As mentioned above, with-condition mortality is not represented directly as a flow in the model, but can be derived as $h_{m_{\text{with}}} = h_m + h_f$.

There are large differences in disease parameters such as incidence and prevalence as a function of age, and it is essential for a model to take this into account. Congenital abnormalities all have a birth prevalence, while important diseases such as dementia and Alzheimer's disease have effectively zero prevalence in the young and dramatically increasing incidence and prevalence at older ages. Furthermore, the incidence and prevalence of disease, as well as the remission and excess mortality hazards, change over time due to shifts in population, changes in prevention or treatment, and changes in care. And the interdependence between these factors is complex but cannot be ignored: today's population of 50-year-olds will be next year's 51-year-olds.

As we will see in the application section, the system of partial differential equations describing the change in the size of the compartments as a function of age and time provides a sufficiently rich theoretical framework for the model of process to integrate all the epidemiological data collected in systematic review. In this formulation, the incidence, remission, without-condition mortality hazard, and excess mortality hazard are all functions of time and age, and the initial conditions for the stock of susceptible and with-condition populations at age 0 are functions of time.

7.3   Endemic equilibrium

The full model is often more complex than can be supported by available data. In order to simplify the modeling procedure and reduce the computational challenge of estimation, it is assumed that the disease parameters do not change substantially with respect to time (in other words, is in endemic equilibrium, to use the jargon of mathematical epidemiology, or is stationary, according to the jargon of time-series analysis). To be precise, this is the assumption that the partial derivative of all stocks and all flows with respect to time is 0:

$$\frac{\partial S}{\partial t} = \frac{\partial C}{\partial t} = \frac{\partial h_i}{\partial t} = \frac{\partial h_r}{\partial t} = \frac{\partial h_m}{\partial t} = \frac{\partial h_f}{\partial t} = 0.$$

Although the primary use of this model is for inference of model parameters (sometimes called the "inverse problem"), it is instructive to apply it to the "forward problem" to show how hazards on incidence, remission, and excess mortality produce different prevalence curves. The next section explores this forward simulation through a series of examples to develop an intuition about how consistency forces interrelationships among prevalence, incidence, remission, and mortality.

7.4   Forward simulation examples

This section begins with a classic example from the history of generic disease modeling, the hypothetical example used in describing DisMod in the first GBD study.[27] The incidence hazard increases linearly from age 0 to 100, and the remission and excess mortality hazards are constant with respect to age. Using all-cause mortality data from Southern sub-Saharan Africa and a birth prevalence of 0 to specify the forward simulation produces the outputs shown in Figure 7.4.

When the age pattern of excess mortality changes to also linearly increase as a function of age, the prevalence curve becomes more clearly nonlinear, showing a condition that increases in prevalence quickly in young age groups but more slowly at older ages. Figure 7.5, panel (a), shows the results of this change.

Although the prevalence age pattern is largely determined by the remission, incidence, and mortality hazards, the birth prevalence can also change the shape dramatically. Figure 7.5, panel (b), shows the results of the same

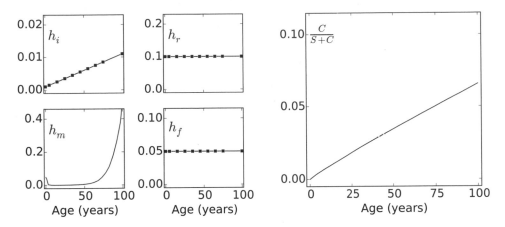

Figure 7.4. Consistent disease parameters for a condition where incidence h_i increases linearly as a function of age while remission h_r and excess mortality h_f hazards are constant. The background mortality h_m has an age-specific hazard that follows all-cause mortality for females in the Southern sub-Saharan region in 1990. For a condition with prevalence of 0 at age 0, these hazards lead to a nearly linear increase as a function of age.

remission, incidence, and mortality hazards as in panel (a), but with a birth prevalence of 1.5%.

To summarize, this series of figures has shown the intuitive and less-than-intuitive way that the levels and age patterns of different epidemiological parameters must be interrelated to satisfy the fundamental equations of population health (when disease hazards for each age change negligibly slowly as a function of time).

Figure 7.6 is designed to continue building familiarity with the features of consistent disease modeling by selecting age patterns for certain hazards to provide stylized examples similar to a variety of diseases. For example, for a disorder like dysthymia, for which there is a minimum duration of 2–3 years and low excess mortality, the consistency conditions produce a prevalence age pattern that looks like a smoothed version of the incidence age pattern, as shown in panel (a). For a congenital disorder, like Down syndrome, with birth prevalence, no incidence after birth, no remission, and substantial mortality, the consistent prevalence age pattern is shown in panel (b). For a disorder that affects the elderly, like Parkinson's disease, the consistent age patterns for mortality, incidence, remission, and prevalence could look roughly like the age-specific rates shown in panel (c). And for disorders related to reproductive health, like uterine prolapse, with zero excess mortality, incidence during ages 15–50, and remission that increases substantially at age 50, the consistent age patterns could look like those shown in panel (d). To conclude this series of plots, I have included an "incidence impulse response" example, showing the prevalence produced to be consistent with an incidence pattern that is nonzero for only a single age group. This is the content of panel (e).

7.5   Summary and future work

This chapter developed the compartmental model for disease moving through a population, which is the key to incorporating data from different epidemiological parameters (e.g., prevalence and incidence).

Future work must focus on the restriction to consider only the endemic equilibrium model of disease. This is justified in many cases and is required in many more. However, there will be applications moving forward where disease rates are changing quickly over time and data are available to demonstrate this. In these cases, it will be necessary to solve the inverse problem without making the endemic equilibrium assumption, which will be a computational challenge.

The focus of the GBD 2010 study led to a prioritization of prevalence estimation from this process, but in other settings it may be other parameters that are of primary interest. For example, age-specific incidence is very important for planning preventive interventions, and age-specific remission rates are important for evaluating a treatment. It is also possible that the general methods here would be of use for more demographic research, where data on all-cause mortality is to be integrated, without attention to a specific disease or risk factor.

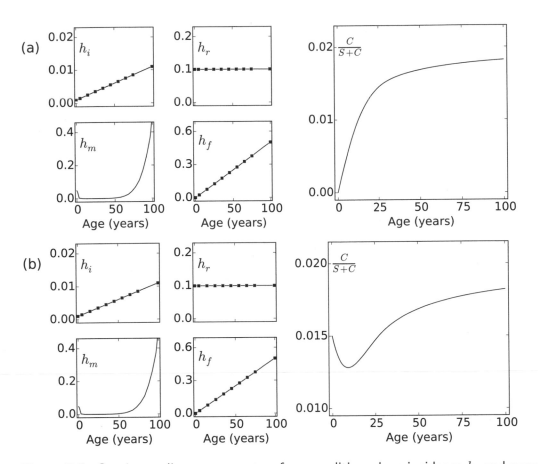

Figure 7.5. Consistent disease parameters for a condition where incidence h_i and excess mortality h_f both increase linearly as a function of age while remission h_r is constant. The background mortality h_m has an age-specific hazard corresponding to females in the Southern sub-Saharan Africa region in 1990. Panel (a) shows that for a condition with prevalence of 0 at age 0, these hazards drive a prevalence age pattern that increases quickly in younger age groups and more slowly in older age groups. Panel (b) shows that for a condition with prevalence of 1.5% at age 0, these rates yield a prevalence age pattern that is highly nonlinear, dipping to a minimum of 1.3% at age 9 and then increasing back up to 1.8% at the oldest ages.

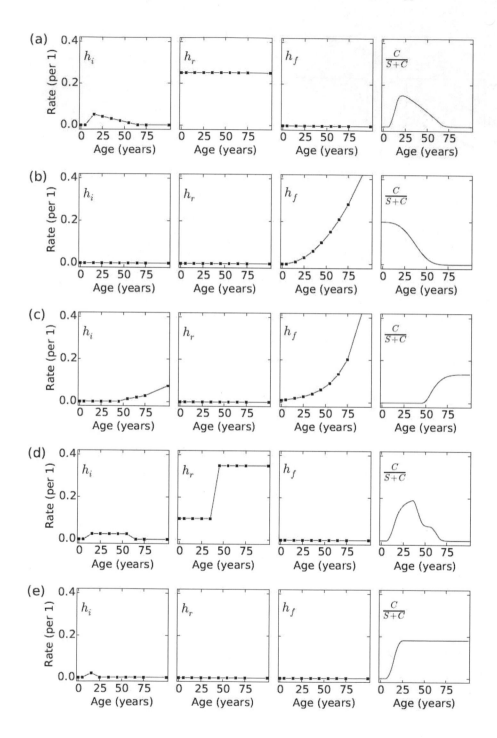

Figure 7.6. Examples of different age-specific rates and the resulting prevalence curves

Chapter 8

Numerical algorithms

Abraham D. Flaxman

Computational tractability has an important influence on model development, which often goes unacknowledged. The models that I fit are a compromise between models I would like to fit and the limitations of the algorithms and computing infrastructure available. This has always been the case, but modern algorithms and modern computing have shifted the balance tremendously.

This chapter will explore the methods that I have used to fit models with the computer. The word algorithm is derived from the name of the medieval mathematician al-Khwarizmi, who developed a precise set of instructions for performing arithmetic with Arabic numerals. Its meaning today is inspired by this. An algorithm a set of instructions so precise that they can be translated into code that a computer can execute. Like al-Khwarizmi's original, the algorithms in this chapter are *numerical*, in the sense that they are concerned with manipulating numbers. This is an area that has received its own name because of some unexpected challenges in attempting to manipulate numbers with digital computers. The binary architecture of the computer is not able to represent the infinite precision of the real numbers from calculus class, and a whole discipline of specialists has grown to cope with this. However, our story begins before this.

In the days before digital computers, computational tractability meant that models had to be simple and computational methods elegant. In the 18th century, for example, an important challenge in predictive modeling was in navigation.[82] Forecasting the path of stars allowed a ship to chart its course accordingly. The method of least squares, first published at the start of that century by Legendre, elegantly provided a solution.[83] Using this method, mathematician-astronomers could plot the location of a celestial body at different time points, postulate a parametric model (e.g., that the the body moves in a straight line), and then use the method of least squares to determine the parameters of the model that best fit the data. Why minimize the squared sum of the residuals? Why not minimize a different distance between the data and a proposed solution? Why not minimize the sum of the distance and the number of parameters in the model? The method of least squares has some appealing theoretical properties, since it is equivalent to finding parameters of maximum likelihood if the errors are normally distributed. But more important, minimizing the squared sum was a computational challenge well matched to the computational resource limitations of the 18th century. It was within reason to calculate the solution with pen and paper.

With the development of digital computation, more computationally intensive methods have become feasible. Topologist Stanislaw Ulam sparked the development of one such class of methods when he challenged himself to calculate the probability of winning in a variant of solitaire in the 1940s. An analytic solution was elusive, but a computationally intensive approximation method gave an approximate solution trivially, at least in theory. Ulam realized that it was more practical to repeat the solitaire game many times and count the number of successful plays than to estimate by pure combinatorial calculations. This approach has grown into the Monte Carlo method, a class of computational methods that rely on repeated random sampling to approximate calculations that are intractable or even impossible to calculate exactly.[84]

The successors to the Monte Carlo algorithm make the Bayesian methods I use in integrative systems modeling possible. In Bayesian terms, the model of process and the model of data articulated in the previous chapters provide a prior distribution and likelihood. In principle, it is a simple application of Bayes' formula to go from this to the posterior distribution. The exact computation of the distribution is intractable for most models of interest, however, and it is algorithms for sampling from the posterior distribution (or a close approximation thereof) that produce the parameter estimates for my models.

Bayesian methods were developed contemporaneously to the method of least squares but were limited in application before the development of Markov chain Monte Carlo (MCMC) algorithms and modern computers. Prior to these innovations, analysis was tractable for only a limited class of prior distributions and likelihoods. But with sufficient computing power, the posterior distribution can be sampled using Monte Carlo methods instead of being computed analytically.[37] Monte Carlo methods can also be applied to integrate the posterior distribution to obtain, for instance, the posterior mean and variance. As computational resources to apply the approach to more complex problems have become more widely available, the approach has gained popularity.[36]

The integrative systems model of disease in a population does not admit a closed-form representation for its posterior distribution. Instead, it relies on MCMC to draw samples of the model parameters from their posterior distribution. This, too, requires some care. The statistical computation tradition has put much effort into deriving Gibbs samplers for specific Bayesian models,[85,86] while theoretical computer scientists have focused on developing generic algorithms like the "Ball Walk" for sampling from convex sets.[87,88] The Metropolis-Hastings step method[89,90,91] and the Adaptive Metropolis (AM) variant,[92] in practice, provide acceptable performance without requiring burdensome derivation of customized Gibbs distributions. The MCMC algorithm benefits from wisely chosen initial values, and this seems to be particularly true when using MCMC with the AM step method in a large parameter space. Powell's method optimizes a function of many variables without requiring derivatives, to find initial values for the model parameters for MCMC.[93] Normal approximation at this initial value finds initial values for the variance-covariance matrices in the AM step method. Furthermore, an empirical Bayes approach separates the global model into submodels that can be fitted in parallel. The remainder of this chapter describes each aspect of the numerical algorithm in more detail.

8.1 Markov chain Monte Carlo

Markov chain Monte Carlo (MCMC) is a class of Monte Carlo methods that obtain approximate solutions using a carefully designed Markov chain. A Markov chain is a stochastic process, or a sequence of random variables, such that the probability distribution of a random variable at one point in the sequence depends only on the random variable immediately before it in the sequence. If a Markov chain satisfies certain conditions, then it must tend toward a unique stationary distribution as the sequence continues. The key to using the MCMC algorithm for integrative systems modeling is constructing a Markov chain with the following three properties:

1. The stationary distribution of the chain is equal to the posterior distribution of the model.

2. Each step of the chain can be computed efficiently.

3. The chain converges to its stationary distribution in a reasonable number of steps.

A simple example can make this clearer. Suppose one wants to sample uniformly from the unit ball in n dimensions, meaning the set of points $\{x \in \mathbb{R}^n : \|x\| \leq 1\}$. The MCMC approach starts from any point in the ball, for example, the origin $X_0 = (0, \ldots, 0)$, and generates successive points $X_1, X_2, \ldots$, randomly, so that the points are Markovian, which is to say that the probability density of X_{i+1} is dependent only on the value of X_i. There is great art to designing the probability density that produces X_{i+1}. In this case, the random scan Gibbs step is a simple one: choose an axis e_i uniformly from the basis $\{e_1, e_2, \ldots, e_n\}$, and then choose X_{i+1} uniformly from the interval given by the intersection of the ball with the line parallel to e_i that passes through X_i.

To be precise, this Markov chain has transition probability density given by

$$\mathbf{p}(X_{i+1} = x | X_i) = \begin{cases} \frac{1}{n} \cdot \frac{1}{2\sqrt{1 - \sum_{j \neq d} x_j^2}}, & \|x\| \leq 1 \text{ and } x_j = X_{i,j} \text{ for all } j \neq d; \\ 0, & \text{otherwise.} \end{cases}$$

When $n = 2$, it is possible to visualize this example in two dimensions, as shown in Figure 8.1.

To see that the uniform distribution of the chain is stationary requires a small calculation. What is the probability density of a point $x \in \mathbb{R}^n$ after a single step of the chain? If $\mathbf{p}(X_i = x) = 1/Z$ for all x, with the notation

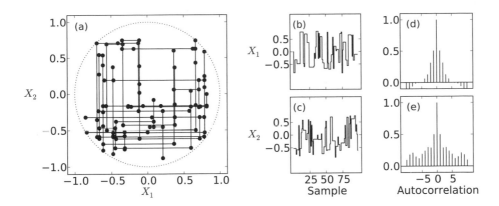

Figure 8.1. The results of drawing 100 samples from a ball in two dimensions with MCMC using the Gibbs step method. Although each sample is dependent on the previous samples, this dependence quickly decays, as shown by plotting the autocorrelation function of $X_1(t)$ and $X_2(t)$ in panels (d) and (e).

$\ell_d = \sqrt{1 - \sum_{j\neq d} x_j^2}$, we have

$$\mathbf{p}(X_{i+1} = x) = \int \int \cdots \int \mathbf{p}(X_{i+1} = x|X_i = x')\mathbf{p}(X_i = x')\mathrm{d}x_1'\mathrm{d}x_2'\cdots\mathrm{d}x_n'$$

$$= \sum_{d=1}^{n} \int \mathbf{p}\left(X_{i+1} = x|X_i = (x_1, \ldots, x_d', \ldots, x_n)\right)$$

$$\times \mathbf{p}\left(X_i = (x_1, \ldots, x_d', \ldots, x_n)\right)\mathrm{d}x_d'$$

$$= \sum_{d=1}^{n} \int_{-\ell_j}^{\ell_j} \frac{1}{n}\frac{1}{2\ell_d}\frac{1}{Z}\mathrm{d}x_d'$$

$$= \frac{1}{Z}.$$

Implementing each step of the chain requires only a way to choose numbers uniformly from the interval $[0, 1]$. This is *not* simple, but it is a basic primitive that randomized computation relies on, and simple-to-use implementations exist, often by default, in modern computer languages; I use the Mersenne Twister pseudorandom number generator, a well-tested standard.[94] To generate X_{i+1} from X_i, the following suffices:

- Choose dimension $d_i \in [n]$ uniformly at random.

- Choose sign $s_i \in \{-1, 1\}$ uniformly at random.

- Choose fraction $f_i \in [0, 1]$ uniformly at random.

- Set X_{i+1} equal to X_i for all coordinates besides d_i and let

$$X_{i+1}(d_i) = s_i f_i \sqrt{1 - \sum_{j \neq d_i} X_i(j)^2}.$$

Proving that Markov chains such as this one rapidly converge to their stationary distributions is a topic of current research in probability theory.

8.2   The Metropolis-Hastings step method

As mentioned above, my approach to parameter estimation with MCMC does *not* rely on deriving Gibbs step methods, which are often much more involved than the simple example in the previous section. I rely heavily on the Metropolis-Hastings (MH) step method and an adaptive variant thereof.[89,90,91]

In the context of Bayesian statistics, the MH algorithm is a technique used to sample from the posterior distribution when the posterior distribution cannot be easily sampled from directly. The algorithm generates the next position of its random walk in two steps. First, it makes a proposal by choosing from a proposal probability distribution, which depends on the current value of the walk. Second, it accepts or rejects this proposal with a probability carefully designed to yield the desired stationary distribution.

In the example from the previous section, uniform sampling from the unit ball, the proposal distribution could be a normal distribution centered at the current value, for example,

$$P_i \sim \text{Normal}\left(X_i, C^2\right).$$

The MH rejection rule is based on the quantity $p_i = \min\left(1, \frac{\mathbf{p}(P_i)\mathbf{p}'(P_i|X_i)}{\mathbf{p}(X_i)\mathbf{p}'(X_i|P_i)}\right)$, where $\mathbf{p}(\cdot)$ is the posterior probability density for value x, and $\mathbf{p}'(p, x)$ is the probability density of proposing p when the chain has value x. The rejection rule is

$$X_{i+1} = \begin{cases} P_i, & \text{with probability } p_i; \\ X_i, & \text{with probability } 1 - p_i. \end{cases}$$

When sampling from the unit ball with the symmetric proposal distribution above, this simplifies to

$$X_{i+1} = \begin{cases} P_i, & \text{if } \|P_i\| \leq 1; \\ X_i, & \text{otherwise.} \end{cases}$$

Making the example from the previous section only a little bit more complicated demonstrates both the utility and the challenges of the MH step method for MCMC. Instead of sampling from the unit ball, now I will consider sampling uniformly from an ellipsoid in n dimensions, $\{x \in \mathbb{R}^n : x^T \Lambda x \leq 1\}$. In this case, the Gibbs step method requires solving a system of equations at each step to determine the limits of the ellipse along the selected dimension. The MH step method requires only testing whether the proposed point is in the ellipse. On the other hand, the Gibbs step method always moves to a new point in the sample space, while MH sometimes rejects the proposal and stays at the same point for multiple steps. In either case, if the ellipse is long and skinny, it will slow the chain. The Gibbs steps will not move very far much of the time, while the MH steps will often not move at all.

When $n = 2$, it is possible to visualize this example in two dimensions, and Figure 8.2 shows the results for an ellipse with width three times its height. It is possible to adjust the proposal distribution to make the chain accept more proposals, and this sort of tuning is an important part of applied MCMC. However, simply shrinking the radius of the ball used to draw proposals will never yield a step method that exploits the correlation between X_1 and X_2; this sort of tuning is the topic of the next section.

8.3 The Adaptive Metropolis step method

The Adaptive Metropolis (AM) step method extends the MH step method by adaptively adjusting the variance-covariance matrix for the proposal distribution based on the acceptance rate of the proposals.[92,95] Because the proposal acceptance rate is so important to algorithmic efficiency, a line of research has considered adaptive approaches to proposal distribution selection.[96,97,98,99]

One popular adaptive approach begins with a simplified version of the MH step method above (often called the Metropolis step method), where a proposal is generated at each step

$$P_i \sim \text{Normal}\left(X_i, C_i^2\right),$$

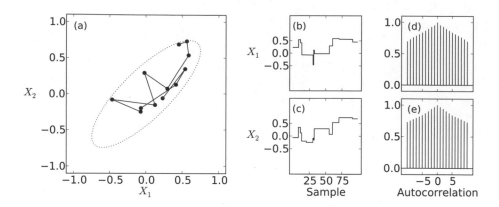

Figure 8.2. The results of drawing 100 samples from an ellipse in two dimensions with MCMC using the MH step method. Each sample is dependent on the previous samples, and because of the shape of the ellipse, the MH proposals are often infeasible, so the dependence does not decay rapidly, as shown by plotting the autocorrelation function of $X_1(t)$ and $X_2(t)$ in panels (d) and (e).

and then accepted or rejected with probability $p_i = \min\left(1, \frac{\mathbf{p}(P_i)}{\mathbf{p}(X_i)}\right)$. This is a simplification of the MH step method, because the terms about the transition probability are not included in the proposal acceptance probability. But it has a subtle complexification of the MH step method as well, because the proposal distribution covariance matrix C_i now changes as the chain progresses. The goal is to change it in a way that adapts to the distribution from which it is being used to sample.

The adaptive values of C_i that I have used follow those implemented in the PyMC software package,[95]

$$C_i = \begin{cases} C_0, & i \le i_0; \\ s_n \left[\text{cov}(X_0, \dots, X_i) + \epsilon I_n\right], & i > i_0. \end{cases}$$

The initial value for the covariance matrix, C_0, has a large influence on the time the MCMC algorithm takes to converge. For the additional parameters, I have used the PyMC default values, where in an n-dimensional sample space, I have used $s_n = (2.4)^2/n$, $\epsilon = 10^{-5}$, and I_n (the n-dimensional identity matrix).

For additional computational speedup, I have followed the PyMC modification of the original AM step method and updated C_i only every 100 or

$1,000$ steps. Furthermore, if few proposals are ever accepted, then I decrease the variance of the proposal distribution by a constant factor.

When $n = 2$, the results of this step method can be visualized in two dimensions, and Figure 8.3 shows the results of the AM stepper after $20,000$ iterations have been run to allow the covariance matrix to adapt to the posterior distribution.

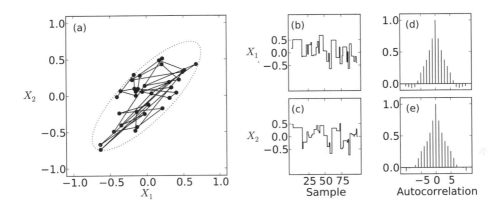

Figure 8.3. The results of drawing 100 samples from an ellipse in two dimensions with MCMC using the AM step method, after $20,000$ iterations of "burn-in." Each sample is dependent on the previous samples, but after a period of exploration, the AM proposals become aligned with the axes of the ellipse, and the dependence decays more rapidly than in the MH approach in Figure 8.2.

8.4   Convergence of the MCMC algorithm

The chief pitfall of the MCMC algorithm is nonconvergence. A line of theoretical research in computer science is devoted to identifying classes of distributions and classes of step methods for which MCMC can be proven to converge rapidly. [87,100,101,102] Unfortunately, this work has recently developed strong evidence against the possibility of automatically detecting convergence of MCMC in general. [103] This work has developed largely separately from that reported in the Bayesian computing literature, where posterior estimates generated by MCMC sampling are used frequently in important settings. [104,105,37] In the applied statistical literature, MCMC is too convenient not to be used, and since nonconvergence is such an important pitfall, a vast array of heuristic checks for convergence have developed over the years. A recent survey compared and contrasted many of these. [106]

Essential to using MCMC for statistical estimation is reproducibility, and here is where nonconvergence wreaks its havoc. MCMC computation is randomized computation, meaning that the same algorithm run on the same data twice will give slightly different answers. This is fine, as long as the variation between successive runs can be controlled. When MCMC has not converged, the difference between two runs cannot be predicted, which means that the results will not be reproducible. This must be prevented for MCMC computation to be useful.

One heuristic to identify nonconvergence that has been particularly useful in my work is to visually inspect the autocorrelation plot for each dimension of the sample space. This autocorrelation function is defined by

$$\mathrm{acf}(\tau) = \frac{\mathbf{E}\left[(X_i - \mu)(X_{i+\tau} - \mu)\right]}{\sigma^2},$$

where μ and σ are the mean and standard deviation of the posterior distribution. The autocorrelation plot for independent samples is a delta function, and the rate of decay of the autocorrelation plot gives some indication of how close the samples are to being uncorrelated. Panels (d) and (e) in Figures 8.1, 8.2, and 8.3 show autocorrelation plots in a provably rapidly mixing chain (Figure 8.1), in a clearly nonconvergent case (Figure 8.2), and in a marginal case that I would run longer to be sure (Figure 8.3).

There are three general approaches to improve the convergence of MCMC computation. The first and simplest approach is to run the chain longer and thus take more samples. In the long run, the algorithm will succeed, and the only question is whether the program can run for long enough in the time available for the analysis. The second approach is to use a more appropriate step method—for example, by using AM steps instead of the MH steps in the ellipse example above. Other, more complicated step methods can also be used, and the development of new and improved step methods is an active area of research. The third approach is to use better initial values for the MCMC, which includes both starting from a likely point in the posterior distribution and, in the case of AM and other advanced step methods, initializing the step method parameters wisely as well. Normalizing model variables is a simple approach that can also help.

The wise selection of initial values is the topic of the next section.

8.5 Initial values for MCMC

Past research has found that the choice of initial values for MCMC can dramatically affect the time necessary for convergence. In theoretical work, a "warm start" increases performance by selecting initial values that are near the target values. Ideally, warm-start values are from a distribution where the density at any point is at most twice the density of the target distribution.[107,108] In practice, a number of different methods have been proposed for generating initial values for MCMC samples.[109,110,111,112,113] The simplest approach is to choose initial values from the prior distribution, either as the expected value of the prior distribution or a random realization of it. In my experience, this is not as stable as choosing initial values based on the results of a local optimization procedure that finds an initial value that approximately maximizes the posterior distribution.

I use a combination of coordinate descent and Powell's method to find a local maximum of the posterior distribution that I then use as the initial values for MCMC.[114,93] In addition to finding a good initial point in the sample space, it is also helpful to find a good initial value for the covariance matrices of the AM step methods. To do this, I use the normal approximation at the maximum posterior, which seems to work well in practice.

8.6 A meta-analysis example

To bring all of these points together, I will now work through a simple example, which we have already seen in the Introduction and Section 1.1: the meta-analysis of five surveys of adult smoking prevalence in the US in 2010. The Bayesian formulation of the fixed effect meta-analysis from Section 1.1 was

$$p_i \sim \text{Normal}(\pi, \sigma_i^2),$$

where π has an uninformative prior, and i ranges over the five nationally representative surveys. In Section 1.1, we derived the posterior distribution of π analytically using Bayes' law. Now let us consider how MCMC would approximate the same result. Suppose we start the chain with $\pi(0)$ equal to the median of the measured prevalences, i.e., the NHIS value of 19.3. From here, the Metropolis step method proposes a perturbed point as the next step, in this case 19.26, and accepts or rejects according to the ratio of the posterior

densities. Table 8.1 shows 10 steps taken in this way and whether they were
accepted or rejected.

Table 8.1. Ten steps with the Adaptive Metropolis (AM) step method for fixed effect
meta-analysis of US smoking prevalence for 2010.

i	π_i	π_i'	$\log \mathbf{p}(\pi_i')$	$\log \pi(p \mid \pi_i')$	$\log \mathbf{p}(\pi_i' \mid p))$	
0		19.30	-4.61	-1982.42	-1987.02	
1	19.30	19.26	-4.61	-1934.30	-1938.91	
2	19.26	19.35	-4.61	-2048.72	-2053.32	rejected
3	19.26	19.64	-4.61	-2444.82	-2449.43	rejected
4	19.26	19.53	-4.61	-2285.01	-2289.62	rejected
5	19.26	19.41	-4.61	-2121.14	-2125.74	rejected
6	19.26	19.50	-4.61	-2245.46	-2250.06	rejected
7	19.26	19.45	-4.61	-2182.36	-2186.96	rejected
8	19.26	19.01	-4.61	-1656.85	-1661.46	
9	19.01	19.27	-4.61	-1947.51	-1952.12	rejected
10	19.01	19.18	-4.61	-1841.50	-1846.11	rejected

As described in Section 8.5, it is helpful to start at a point $\pi(0)$ that has a
relatively high posterior probability density. In this case, a chain started from
an unlikely point quickly converges to a likely point, and the AM step method
is not relevant because the model has a single scalar parameter. The tuning
of the proposal distribution is relevant, however. With too large a proposal
distribution, the chain will rarely accept, and with too small a proposal distribution the chain will accept frequently but not move very much. In either
case, the autocorrelation function will decay slowly.

8.7 Empirical Bayesian priors to borrow strength between regions

When making estimates for all 21 geographic regions in the GBD 2010 study,
the available data were often very sparse. I have often used an approach
to borrow strength between regions. It is a two-stage approach that can be
characterized as an empirical Bayesian technique.

The mechanics of this approach are simple. First, I fit a model to the
available data at the global level. Depending on the data available, this is

often either an inconsistent model, using the random-effect age-integrating negative-binomial spline model from Chapters 3–6, or a consistent model linking random-effect age-integrating negative-binomial spline models for different epidemiological parameters through the system of differential equations in Section 7.2. This model is used to make estimates for all regions of the world.

The second stage of the empirical Bayes approach is to use the first-stage predictions for a region as priors and to fit the model again, now including the empirical priors, with only the data relevant to a particular region, sex, and year.

There is a well-founded philosophical objection to this approach. An appeal of the Bayesian way is its theoretical foundation, which requires using data precisely once when going from priors to posteriors. On the other hand, as a practical matter the computation necessary to avoid the empirical Bayes approach is not tractable in some cases, and here the two-stage approach can be interpreted as an approximation to a fully Bayesian hierarchical model. This approximation uses the same data twice, which leads to an underestimate of the width of uncertainty intervals, and could potentially produce a substantial underestimate. Investigating this further is sure to be a fruitful area for future work, and we will return to the implications of this method in a specific example in Chapter 11.

8.8 Summary and future work

The MCMC algorithm, with the AM step method, has been an enabler for this entire approach. Without free/libre open-source software for implementing AM/MCMC[95] the DisMod-MR project would not have been possible. Initial values from optimization of the posterior distribution and the empirical prior approach to decompose the regional estimation tasks into independent calculations were also crucial to finding reasonable answers in the available computation time.

A new approach to MCMC step methods, based on automatic computation of the gradient of the posterior distribution, is one direction for speeding the process of fitting these models. Hamiltonian Monte Carlo and the No U-Turn Sampler are two examples of this approach that seem particularly worthy of future investigation.[56,57]

However, this MCMC-based computation is not the only algorithmic approach. Message-passing algorithms have proven themselves quite successful in related computational challenges[115,116], and variational approaches are also promising.[117] Nonlinear optimization is another promising approach, especially combined with the bootstrap method for estimating uncertainty.[118] As computational resources continue to evolve and new computational algorithms are developed, the possibility of incorporating innovations into faster and more accurate estimates should be continually explored.

8.9   Challenges and limitations

The computation time necessary to fit this model is one of the most important challenges in its routine use. Alternative models for spatial pooling, modeling temporal trends, and a routine method for conducting out-of-sample cross-validation are other areas where there is room for further research. The book turns now to example applications of this model to a range of disease and risk factor estimation tasks, and will return to challenges, limitations, and areas for future work in more detail in Chapter 20.

Part II

Applications

The application portion of this book contains a range of examples taken from the GBD 2010 study. These examples are designed to match and clarify the model features developed in the theory and methods portion of the book. It is quite possible to browse the application chapters, as they do not rely on each other, and to make it easy for readers to identify applications matching their particular interests, the following table describes each application briefly and indicates to which part of the theory and methods section it is matched.

Application chapters in the applications section

Application Chapter	Condition	Demonstrates	Theory Chapter
9	Cocaine dependence	Spline modeling and knot selection for sparse and noisy data	3.1-3.4
10	Premenstrual syndrome	Expert priors on age patterns for sparse and noisy data	4
11	Pancreatitis	Empirical priors to borrow strength between countries and regions when necessary	4.4, 8.7
12	Atrial fibrillation	Age-standardizing to combine data for heterogeneous age groups	5
13	Hepatitis C virus	Spatial random effects to capture variation within and between countries and regions	6.4
14	Anxiety disorders	Cross-walk fixed effects to combine measurements with different diagnostic criteria	6.1
15	Liver cirrhosis	Predictive fixed effects for more accurate out-of-sample estimation	6.2

Application chapters (continued)

Application Chapter	Condition	Demonstrates	Theory Chapter
16	Fruit consumption	Log-normal likelihood for a continuous exposure variable	2
17	End-stage renal disease	Using the compartmental model to integrate different types of epidemiological data	7.2
18	Osteoarthritis of the knee	Knot selection in compartmental models	3.2, 7.2
19	Bipolar disorder	Expert priors in compartmental models	4, 7.2
20	Alcohol dependence	Using cause-specific mortality rate data as a lower bound in the compartmental model	7.2

Chapter 9

Knot selection in spline models: cocaine dependence

Yong Yi Lee, Theo Vos, Abraham D. Flaxman, Jed Blore, and Louisa Degenhardt

For many conditions, prevalence varies substantially as a function of age. Other epidemiological parameters, such as incidence and excess mortality hazards, often have important age patterns as well. The spline models introduced in Chapter 3 provide a flexible framework for representing this age dependence. However, some important modeling decisions are necessary. The following examples from estimating the age-specific prevalence of cocaine dependence illustrate the importance of choosing knot locations and smoothing levels appropriately in a setting where the data speak relatively precisely about the level and age pattern of the condition.

The American Psychiatric Association's *Diagnostic and Statistical Manual of Mental Disorders, Version IV, Text Revision (DSM-IV-TR)* recognizes cocaine dependence as fulfilling three or more of the following seven dependence criteria during any time in the same 12-month period:[119,120]

- tolerance to effects of cocaine (typically assessed by whether the same amount of cocaine has less effect or whether greater amounts are required to obtain the desired effect);

- withdrawal symptoms after use ceases;

- usage over a longer period or in larger quantities than intended;

- persistent desire or unsuccessful efforts to control cocaine use;

- substantial time spent in obtaining, using, or recovering from effects of cocaine;

- reduction of important social, occupational, or recreational activities because of cocaine use;

- continued use despite knowledge of physiological or psychological problems induced by cocaine use.

Despite a large body of data on cocaine *use*, there are comparatively few data available on the descriptive epidemiology of cocaine *dependence*.[121] Systematic review for cocaine dependence identified 28 prevalence data points, covering three GBD 2010 regions. For this example, we have restricted our attention to data from the US (Figure 9.1).

As discussed in Chapter 3, we model age-specific hazards with spline models. In this case, the spline model takes the form of a continuous, piecewise linear function, with knots, selected as part of the model, where the function is nonlinear. The knots partition the age range into intervals, and the choice of knots can be influential for the resulting estimates. In a setting where data are *not* sparse, estimates will not be very sensitive to the choice of knots. However, when working with sparse data, the number and location of knots are important decisions, as they can influence the model results substantially. Ideally, the number and locations of knots should be chosen a priori, based on expert knowledge of the disease being modeled. It is also a good practice to consider additional knots and alternative configurations of knots as a sensitivity analysis. A unique aspect of knot selection in metaregression is the way the heterogeneous age intervals and knots interact. The subtlety of this interaction can produce estimates with more certainty than is warranted.

To demonstrate the effect of the number and location of knots in a spline model, we compare three choices of knots in Figure 9.2. The 4-knot model for cocaine dependence has knots at $0, 14, 15$, and 100, and jumps from a prevalence of zero at young ages (a model assumption enforced by a level value prior based on the theory that prevalence is zero in childhood and changes rapidly during early adulthood) to a prevalence of 7 per 1,000 at age 15. From there, the prevalence decreases gradually as age increases, with a linear age pattern because the spline model has no knots between ages 15 and 100.

The 5-knot model has knots at $0, 14, 25, 35$, and 100. The estimates from this model, shown as a dotted line, rise to a peak of 14 per 1,000 at age 25, and then fall off, faster from age 25 to 35 than after age 35.

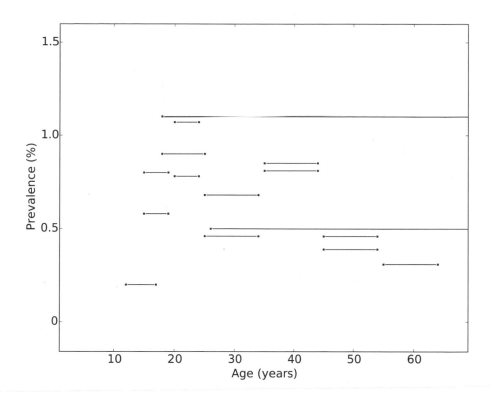

Figure 9.1. Prevalence data for cocaine dependence in the US. Each horizontal bar represents a single data point extracted in systematic review. The left and right endpoints indicate the start and end ages of the age interval for a data point, while the level of prevalence is represented by the distance of the bar above the x-axis.

The 8-knot model has knots at $0, 15, 20, 25, 30, 40, 50$, and 100. The estimates from this model are shown as a dashed line in Figure 9.2. For these knots, the model estimates are able to follow the bimodal pattern in the data, peaking at 13 per 1,000 at age 20, and then falling and rising again before tapering off.

If the differing choices of ages 14 and 15 for the second knot in the models above disturbs you, that is good; it should. This modeling choice has implications for the estimates generated and should not be made arbitrarily. One principled approach is to include additional knots, so that when the data

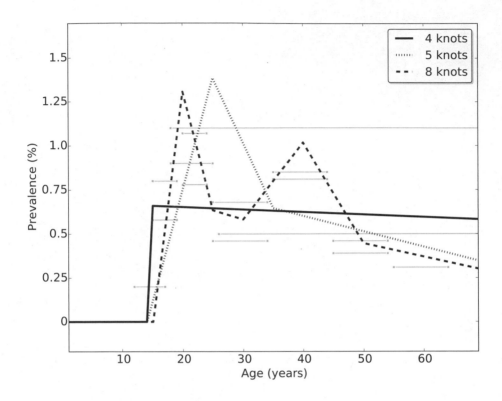

Figure 9.2. Prevalence estimates of cocaine dependence in the US using a spline model with 4, 5, and 8 knots.

are insufficient for identifying the minimum age of onset of the condition, at least the model estimates will capture this uncertainty. Panels (a) and (b) of Figure 9.3 compare the 8-knot model above, which contains only one knot between ages 10 and 20, with a model with knots at ages 10, 12, 14, 16, 18, and 20 instead of at age 15 only. This leads to wider uncertainty intervals in the estimates for ages under 20, of course, but it also leads to wider uncertainty intervals for age 25, because the increased flexibility of the age pattern for teens allows the model to consider a wider range of age-specific prevalence for twenty-somethings as well.

This line of inquiry has a natural next step. Why not include additional knots in the older ages as well? The panels (c) and (d) of Figure 9.3 investigate the effects of this. In panel (c), where there are knots every two years from age 10 to age 60, the effects are two-fold: a more wiggly point estimate and wider uncertainty intervals. When the data only refer to broad age intervals, there are many ways for an age pattern to match it, which is just another way to see that the choice of knots matters. Panel (d) shows a pitfall of MCMC methods that was mentioned in Section 8.4, nonconvergence. This model has knots every two years from age 0 to age 100 and has produced an estimate for prevalence at age 60 that is much lower than all other models. This is probably because the posterior distribution for spline knots for ages above 55 has high correlation, which prevents the MCMC random walk from mixing as rapidly as in the other cases.

The computation time required to fit the model increases with the number of knots. For 10,000 iterations of MCMC, the times range from under two minutes for the 4-knot model to over three and a half minutes for the 8-knot model. The model with 51 knots spaced at two-year age intervals takes 57 minutes to go 10,000 iterations but seems to need many times more iterations to produce nearly independent samples from the approximate stationary distribution. Thus, the strategy of adding more knots must be balanced against considerations of computation time and algorithmic convergence.

The penalized spline model from Section 3.3 introduces an additional term to the model prior to encode the belief that the age pattern is not too wiggly. With the judicious choice of the smoothness hyperparameter, the model can include more knots without using them to chase the noise around in the noisy data. The effects of four values of the smoothing parameter are shown in Figure 9.4. The smaller the parameter, the smoother the estimated age pattern and, hence, the less influential the position of the knots. However, too much smoothing leads to overcompression of the prevalence estimates, resulting in estimates that are not representative of the data.

If there were enough time and data, it would be ideal to compare out-of-sample predictive validity for a range of knots and smoothing parameters, although in-sample criteria of model fitness such as the Akaike information criteria (AIC), Bayesian information criteria (BIC), or deviance information criteria (DIC), can also give some idea without requiring additional computation. [122] Table 9.1 compares these model fitness criteria for a range of knots and smoothness parameters.

According to AIC and BIC, the 8-knot model with no smoothing penalty provides the best fit to the data. DIC gives a different assessment, although the large negative numbers for two models may be due to nonconvergence

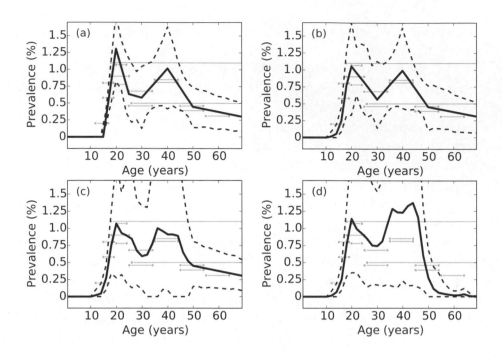

Figure 9.3.   Prevalence estimates of cocaine dependence in the US using a spline model with (a) 8 knots at $0, 15, 20, 25, 30, 40, 50$, and 100; (b) 12 knots at $0, 10, 12, 14, 16, 18, 20, 25, 30, 40, 50$, and 100; (c) 23 knots at $0, 10, 12, \ldots, 48, 50$ and 100; and (d) 51 knots at $0, 2, \ldots, 98, 100$.

rather than fit quality. The 8-knot model with smoothing penalty 0.5 (which we consider "slightly" smooth) is very similar to AIC and BIC fit quality, and produces the estimates shown in Figure 9.3(a).

This chapter has explored how knot location and smoothing penalty selection can be influential parts of the model estimates. In the next chapter, we will consider a related case where the data do not have as clear a story to tell about the age pattern.

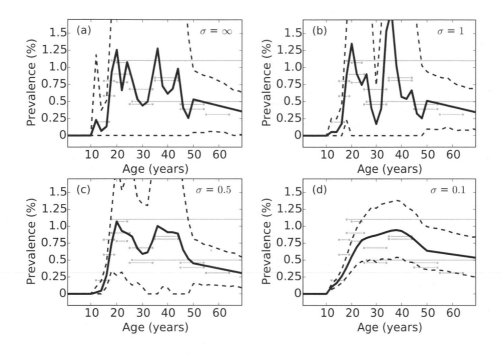

Figure 9.4. Prevalence estimates from the model with knots at $0, 10, 12, \ldots, 48, 50$ and 100 using a penalized spline model with a smoothing parameter $\sigma = \infty, 1, 0.5, 0.1$.

Knot selection in spline models

Table 9.1. Comparison of Akaike information criteria (AIC), Bayesian information criteria (BIC), and deviance information criteria (DIC) goodness-of-fit metrics for a range of knots and smoothness parameters.

Knots	σ	AIC	BIC	DIC
$0, 15, 20, 25, 30, 40, 50, 100$	∞	158	171	132
$0, 15, 20, 25, 30, 40, 50, 100$	1.0	158	171	133
$0, 15, 20, 25, 30, 40, 50, 100$	0.5	159	172	141
$0, 10, 12, 14, 16, 18, 20, 25, 30, 40, 50, 100$	∞	165	182	133
$0, 10, 12, 14, 16, 18, 20, 25, 30, 40, 50, 100$	1.0	165	182	102
$0, 10, 12, 14, 16, 18, 20, 25, 30, 40, 50, 100$	0.5	166	183	141
$0, 10, 12, 14, 16, 18, 20, 25, 30, 40, 50, 100$	0.1	182	199	152
$0, 10, 12, ..., 48, 50, 100$	∞	186	212	-1041
$0, 10, 12, ..., 48, 50, 100$	1.0	187	214	-103
$0, 10, 12, ..., 48, 50, 100$	0.5	188	215	139
$0, 15, 20, 25, 30, 40, 50, 100$	0.1	199	212	182
$0, 10, 12, ..., 48, 50, 100$	0.1	206	232	152

Chapter 10

Unclear age pattern, requiring expert priors: premenstrual syndrome

Hannah M. Peterson, Yong Yi Lee, Theo Vos, and Abraham D. Flaxman

Epidemiological data without clear age patterns are a reoccurring theme in GBD 2010. Although this is occasionally because age is not an important predictor, it is much more often because of the sparse and noisy data available. Unclear age patterns make expert priors essential in the modeling process. However, such cases are very sensitive to the choice of prior assumptions, as shown in the following example of premenstrual syndrome (PMS) in Western Europe.

PMS is a common cyclic disorder that affects women of reproductive years during the time between ovulation and the onset of menses. More than 200 behavioral, psychological, and physical symptoms have been associated with PMS, the most common being irritability, tension, depression, bloating, weight gain, and food cravings. The exact causes of PMS are unknown, with no consistent treatment option available. [123,124,125]

A systematic review of the descriptive epidemiology of PMS yielded 74 prevalence data points, of which 18 were from Western Europe. [6] As seen in Figure 10.1, the data are noisy, with overlapping and heterogeneous age groups that show contradictory age patterns.

In the absence of clear age patterns in the systematic review data points, modeling decisions about knot location, age pattern levels, and direction of age pattern trends have substantial influence on the estimates of disease preva-

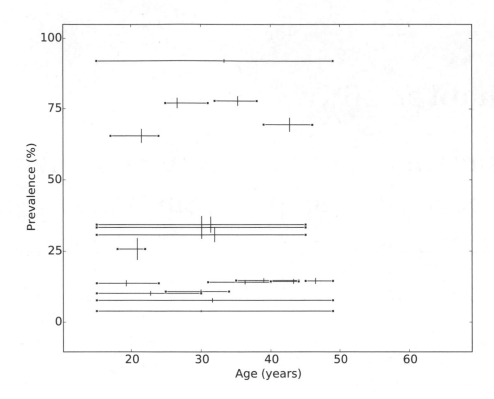

Figure 10.1. Prevalence data for women with PMS in Western Europe. Each horizontal bar represents a single data point extracted in systematic review. The left and right endpoints indicate the start and end ages of the age interval for a data point, while the level of prevalence is represented by the distance of the bar above the x-axis. The vertical bars crossing near the midpoint of each horizontal bar indicate the reported standard error of each measurement.

lence. These decisions can also have unintended consequences, as discussed in Chapter 3. To illustrate the effects, we fitted models with a variety of choices about knot location, level values outside the measured age intervals, and direction of age pattern trends. Conducting a sensitivity analysis like this is important. The sensitivity analysis allows the modeler to understand the range of answers for the given assumptions and provides a long-term guide for identifying areas of future research to collect more precise estimates.

As the prevalence data plotted in Figure 10.1 show, systematic review collected no data on population prevalence for women younger than age 15 or older than age 50. Since PMS is a disorder related to the female reproductive cycle, it follows that data outside this age range are not present for biological reasons. However, this information is not part of the spline model unless the modeler explicitly includes it. If no priors are included to inform estimates in the young and old, then the spline model extrapolates from the levels where there are data, as seen in Figure 10.2. The spline model can start and end at ages appropriate to the analysis and avoid extrapolation altogether, but for the purposes of the GBD 2010 study, estimates for all ages were required; an assumption that the prevalence is zero before age 15 and after age 50 and a truncated analysis within this range is equivalent to strong priors on the level before age 15 and after age 50, provided the spline model has knots at 14, 15, 50, and 51. The sensitivity analysis shown in Figure 10.2 highlights the effect of modeling assumptions; prevalence at ages younger than 15 and older than 50 is biologically implausible, and expert knowledge is needed to inform the model that cases are not expected outside the age range where they have been measured.

As described in Section 3.1 and explored in detail in the previous chapter, we model age-specific hazards with splines, using knots to partition the age range into intervals. Models with ample data and clear age patterns are not very sensitive to knot choice. However, for data without a clear age pattern, the number and location of knots can influence the model results substantially. We explored this by fitting models with a variety of knots to the PMS dataset, as seen in Figure 10.3. As discussed in Chapter 9, choosing the number and location of knots a priori using expert knowledge allows the user to determine critical features of the model in a principled way.

Another common prior for age patterns is the belief that the epidemiological parameter increases or decreases over a certain age range. As seen in Figure 10.4, priors on monotonicity between the critical ages of 25 and 40 have a large effect on the prevalence estimate for Western Europe.

Knot selection and priors on level and monotonicity play an important role in the modeling process and in the sensitivity analysis. However, when the data are not sufficient to understand the age pattern, the model compensates by producing estimates with large uncertainty, as seen in Figure 10.5. This estimate comes from a model with knots at $\{0, 15, 20, 30, 40, 50, 100\}$, no prior on monotonicity, and a prior on level to restrict prevalence to be 0 outside the age range 15–50.

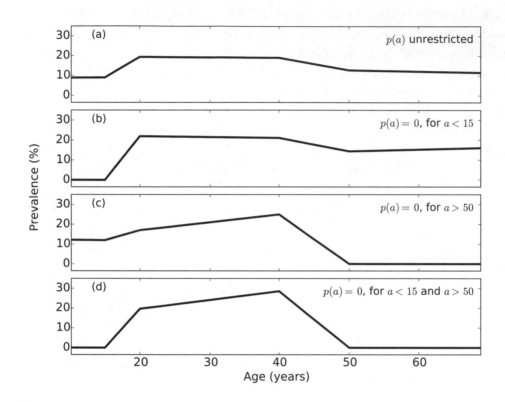

Figure 10.2. Four estimates of age-specific PMS prevalence with different priors on prevalence in young and old ages. Systematic review produced sparse and noisy data, shown here for Western Europe. (a) Without a level prior to inform the model that prevalence data are not present outside ages 15–50 for biological reasons, estimates outside the ages measured are extrapolated from inside. Restricting prevalence to 0 changes the prevalence estimates substantially. (b) The effect of assuming $p(a) = 0$ for $a < 15$, (c) the effect of assuming $p(a) = 0$ for $a > 50$, and (d) the effect of assuming $p(a) = 0$ for $a < 15$ and $a > 50$ all change the estimates inside and outside the observed data ages.

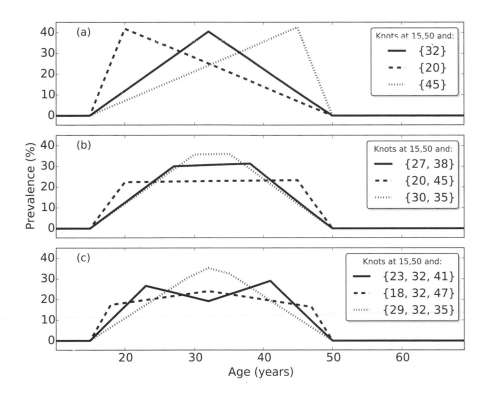

Figure 10.3. Estimate of age-specific PMS prevalence for spline models with a variety of knots. All panels have knots at $\{0, 15, 50, 100\}$ and vary the number and location of knots between the ages of 15 and 50 to show the sensitivity of knot selection in data without a clear age pattern. (a) With one additional knot, the placement at age 20, 32, or 45 gives markedly different estimates of PMS prevalence in Western Europe. (b) With two knots at $\{27, 38\}$, $\{20, 45\}$, or $\{30, 35\}$, the differences are also clear and predictable. (c) With three knots at locations $\{23, 32, 41\}$, $\{18, 32, 47\}$, or $\{29, 32, 35\}$, it appears that the data are too sparse and noisy to support a consistent age pattern.

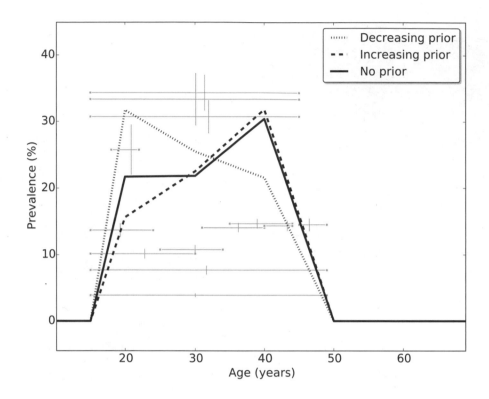

Figure 10.4. Estimates of age-specific PMS prevalence for spline models with a variety of monotonicity priors. Between the ages of 25 and 40, the prior on monotonicity makes a large impact on the prevalence estimates for women in Western Europe with PMS.

This example has identified an area of future research. The model does not have enough data to inform an age pattern because the descriptive epidemiology of PMS is quite uncertain: some studies say almost all women experience it and some studies say none do. In such cases, making the most informed decisions possible (such as restricting the model to ages 15–50 for biological reasons) and accepting a large uncertainty interval reveal the truth: we just don't know.

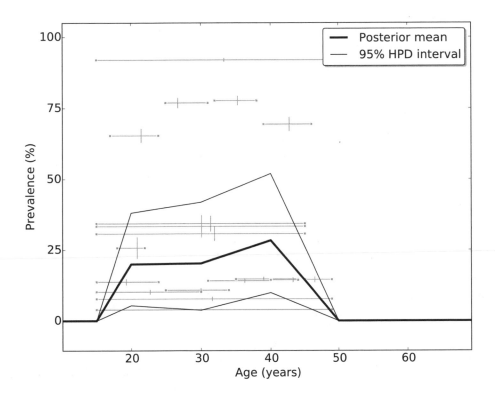

Figure 10.5. Prevalence estimates for women in Western Europe with PMS.

Chapter 11

Empirical priors: pancreatitis

David Chou, Hannah M. Peterson, Abraham D. Flaxman,
Christopher J.L. Murray, and Mohsen Naghavi

Systematic review for GBD 2010 often found a few regions for which detailed data on the age patterns of disease were available, but many more
regions for which cases were reported with much sparser age specificity. Hierarchical modeling using an empirical Bayesian prior is our way to conduct
partial pooling and borrow strength from the regions with age-specific data to
produce estimates of age patterns in regions where few or no age-specific data
are available. This empirical prior approach is a method of convenience, and it
would be philosophically appealing to use a single hierarchical model, instead
of a two-stage approach. This chapter compares results from a single hierarchical model and a two-stage empirical prior for partial pooling at the regional
level, where country-to-country variation is quite pronounced, by examining
the estimation of age-specific pancreatitis incidence in Western Europe.

Pancreatitis is the inflammation of the pancreas, most commonly caused
by alcohol or gallstones. In most cases, the disease resolves itself and there
is no need for treatment. However, some acute cases progress to pancreatic
necrosis and systemic organ failure. These complications require immediate
treatment and have a high mortality risk. [126,127,128]

Data from systematic review yielded 3, 950 incidence data points, 1, 053 of
which were from Western Europe and constitute the example in this chapter.
As shown in Figure 11.1, the data from Western Europe are very noisy, and
the pooled estimates mask heterogeneous age patterns, especially between the
ages of 25 and 60.

Closer investigation of Figure 11.2 shows that the heterogeneity in age patterns reflects between-country variation. The pooled estimate in Figure 11.1

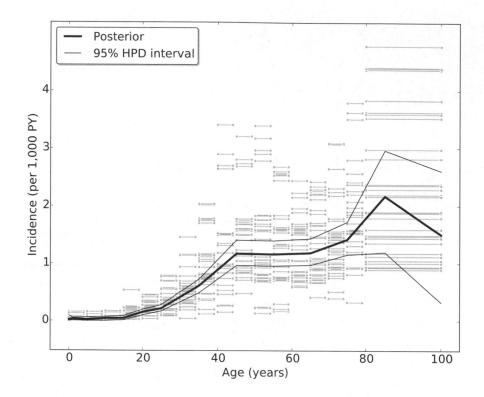

Figure 11.1. Pancreatitis incidence data with pooled estimates for males and females in Western Europe, 2005.

does not capture this age-specific variation. However, country-specific posterior estimates, made with an empirical prior and partial pooling, as described in Section 8.7, can produce estimates that represent this age-specific variation, as shown in Figure 11.2.

When making estimates for a country with an abundance of consistent data, the empirical prior has little influence, and the posterior is informed almost entirely by the data. In a setting where no data are available, the posterior estimate follows the empirical prior with large uncertainty intervals since the countries with data show a lot of country-to-country variation (this large uncertainty is also the reason why the means of the empirical prior and posterior estimates for Germany in panel (d) do not match precisely).

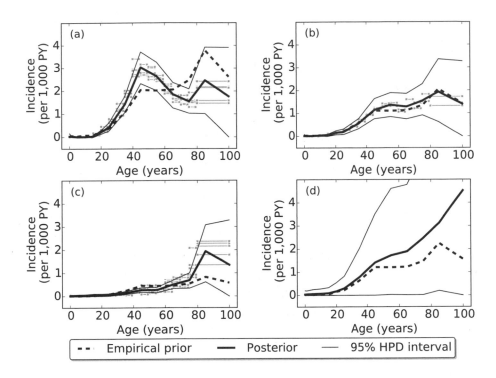

Figure 11.2. Comparison of pancreatitis incidence estimates for males in 2005 for (a) Finland, (b) the Netherlands, (c) Cyprus, and (d) Germany. The estimated incidence using pooled data from Figure 11.1 was applied as an empirical prior to the sex-specific incidence to improve estimates.

As mentioned in Section 8.7, the Bayesian way for data analysis prefers to avoid this two-stage approach to borrowing strength across countries through partial pooling. Instead of following an empirical Bayes approach, it is philosophically preferred to use a hierarchical model that fits age-specific hazard functions for all countries simultaneously.

One way to do this is to employ the hierarchical similarity priors described in Section 4.4. In the notation from that section, this model takes the form:

$$h_i(a) \sim \text{Normal}\left(e^{\alpha_i}\boldsymbol{\mu}(a), \sigma^2\right) \text{ for } a \in A, i \in C;$$
$$\alpha_i \sim \text{Normal}\left(0, \sigma_\alpha^2\right);$$
$$\boldsymbol{\mu}(a) \sim h_{\text{region}}(a);$$
$$\sigma_\alpha \sim \text{TruncatedNormal}_{[0.01,10]}(0.1, 2);$$
$$\sigma(a) \sim \text{TruncatedNormal}_{[0.5,10]}(1, 1^2).$$

This approach does not use the same data twice, and therefore is expected to produce larger uncertainty intervals than the intervals estimated by empirical Bayes. However, the chain takes longer to run and requires more iterations for convergence. After 200,000 iterations (7.5 hours of CPU time), the draws from the posterior distribution were highly correlated even after 1,000 steps of MCMC. As the number of countries and regions in such an analysis increases, we expect that the time required for the MCMC algorithm to converge will increase super-linearly, making it infeasible for general use with the currently available datasets, computers, and algorithms. The hierarchical approach described here has some ad hoc elements as well, and as computational advances make such a method feasible for routine use, there will also be a need for additional modeling work to explore alternative approaches to formulating the hierarchical similarity priors.

Despite the challenges of MCMC convergence and computation time, it is still possible to compare estimates from the hierarchical model and the empirical Bayes model. The posterior distribution for age-standardized pancreatitis incidence in the Netherlands (where some data were available to inform the estimate) is 22% larger in the hierarchical model than the empirical Bayes model.

In summary, empirical priors provide a practical method for partial pooling of data to borrow strength across countries and regions. In cases where data are abundant, this has little impact, while in cases where there are no data, this provides estimates based on the group mean. In cases where some data are available, this approach comes up with something, but the estimates it produces may be more certain than they should be, due to the compromise of the empirical Bayes approach.

Chapter 12

Overlapping, heterogeneous age groups: atrial fibrillation

Mohammad H. Forouzanfar, Abraham D. Flaxman,
Hannah M. Peterson, Mohsen Naghavi, and Sumeet Chugh

Like many conditions analyzed in GBD 2010, atrial fibrillation (AF) has no standard set of age groups for reporting. The meta-analysis of the data collected in systematic review must address these heterogeneous age groups in some way. AF provides a prototypical example of this, one where the results of the choice to use an age-standardizing model can be compared with those of other possible choices. This chapter compares the estimates produced for AF prevalence and incidence using an age-standardizing model with those from a midpoint model.

AF is the most common type of cardiac arrhythmia. Chaotic and irregular heart rhythms originating in the atria cause poor blood flow to the body. The duration of AF episodes varies greatly. Paroxysmal AF is occasional, with attacks lasting a few minutes or hours, whereas persistent AF and permanent AF are chronic, continuing for days with or without self-termination. Symptoms include heart palpitations, lack of energy, dizziness, shortness of breath, and chest discomfort, although some cases of AF are symptomless. AF may occur at any age, with increasing risk for older ages, and is uncommon in children. Other heart diseases tend to be the underlying causes of AF. AF is associated with coronary heart disease, hypertensive heart disease, valvular heart disease, heart failure, cardiomyopathy, obesity, and metabolic disorders such as diabetes and hyperthyroidism.[129,130,131,132]

The GBD 2010 study defines AF as a patient having at least one episode confirmed by a physician. The systematic review of AF collected 3,942 data points, of which 247 were from countries in Western Europe. We will consider only the Western European data in this chapter. We have 20 data points on disease incidence and 147 on prevalence. As seen in Figure 12.1, AF has heterogeneous and overlapping age groups. Without access to the microdata needed to recreate homogeneous age groups, combining all these data must rely on age-group modeling, as described in Chapter 5.

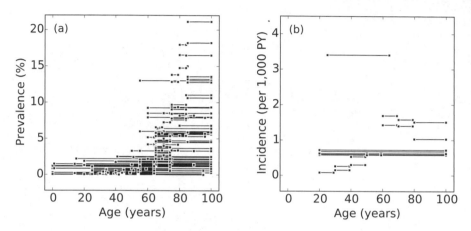

Figure 12.1. Data for prevalence and incidence of AF in Western European males. This is a typical example of the sort of heterogeneous and overlapping age groups collected in systematic review.

As discussed in Section 5.2, the simplest approach to modeling heterogeneous age groups is to apply each age-specific rate measurement to the midpoint of the age interval. Another solution to the heterogeneous age groups is to use age standardizing (Section 5.5). Age standardizing adds age weights to the age-specific rate according to population structure. The age-standardizing model uses a common age pattern for all studies so that the age weights are the same for all country-years, as discussed in more detail in Section 5.5.

As the prevalence estimates in Figure 12.2 show, model choice changes the estimates. In estimates before age 80, differences are minimal, but in estimates for older ages, where the data are sparser and noisier, the differences are substantial.

Without additional information, one cannot say which model is preferred. Further investigation with incidence does not provide much insight. Figure 12.3 shows that, like the prevalence estimates, the incidence estimates

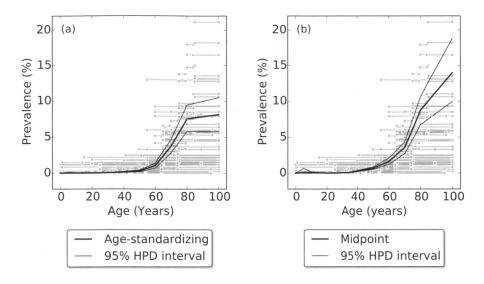

Figure 12.2. Comparison of estimates of prevalence of atrial fibrillation for Western European males in 1990: (a) data and estimates for the age-standardizing model, as described in Section 5.2; (b) data and estimates for the midpoint model (Section 5.5).

are similar in younger ages but are markedly different in older ages. The age-standardizing model also produces estimates with a smoother age pattern.

Using all available data in a compartmental model, including the limited available data on excess mortality, with-condition mortality, and cause-specific mortality, is a way to combine the data on incidence and prevalence to produce internally consistent estimates by modeling all parameters simultaneously. The prevalence estimates from this model are preferred to those from a spline model of prevalence alone because the compartmental model incorporates additional data. Compartmental models are discussed in more detail in Section 7.2. Figure 12.4 shows consistent prevalence and incidence estimates from the age-standardizing compartmental model.

The compartmental model estimates for incidence in Figure 12.4 are very different from the spline model estimates. Unlike the spline models, the compartmental model estimates for incidence do not go through all the data. This is because the compartmental model requires internal consistency; that is, for every prevalence case there must be a matching incidence event. The com-

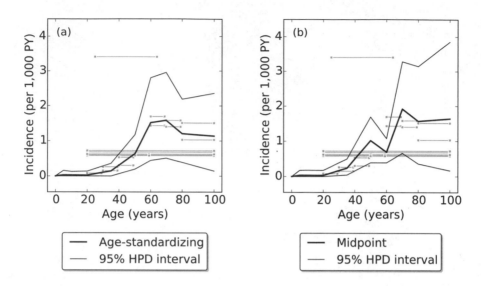

Figure 12.3. Comparison of estimates of incidence of atrial fibrillation for Western European males in 1990: (a) data and estimates for the age-standardizing model; (b) data and estimates for the midpoint model.

partmental model shows that these levels of prevalence cannot be achieved with the levels of incidence the data show.

Figure 12.5 compares the prevalence and incidence estimates from the age-standardizing compartmental model with those from the midpoint compartmental model. As with the spline models, the estimates differ substantially only in the oldest ages.

The choice of age-group model has implications for disease estimates. Estimated age pattern, trends, and levels can differ between the midpoint and age-standardizing models. The age-standardizing model is a unique feature of the approach developed in this book and allows more appropriate use of systematic review data than simply applying the measurement to the midpoint of the age interval.

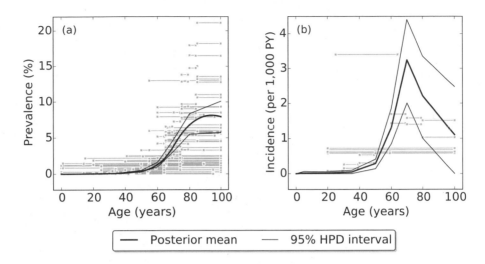

Figure 12.4. Estimates of atrial fibrillation in Western European males in 1990 using an age-standardizing compartmental model for (a) prevalence and (b) incidence.

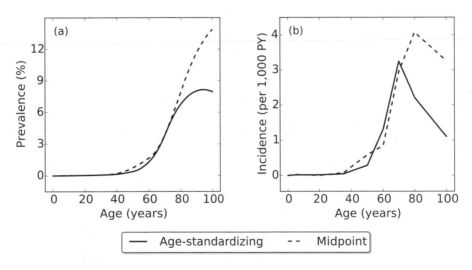

Figure 12.5. Comparison of the estimated (a) prevalence and (b) incidence of atrial fibrillation in Western European males in 1990 using age-standardizing and midpoint compartmental models.

Chapter 13

Dealing with geographical variation: hepatitis C virus infection

Abraham D. Flaxman, Khayriyyah Mohd Hanafiah,
Justina Groeger, Hannah M. Peterson, and Steven T. Wiersma

One challenge in global disease modeling for descriptive epidemiological estimation is properly reflecting the true regional variation in disease epidemiology. While some diseases are relatively consistent in their levels and age patterns from region to region, others vary a great deal. The most extreme examples of the latter type are focal diseases that are present only in certain regions, but the hardest to model are diseases that are present globally, but to greater and lesser degrees. Hepatitis C virus (HCV) is an example of such a disease, which we examine in this chapter. In the absence of any predictive covariates to model with fixed effects, we use hierarchical random effects to model this regional variation.

Hepatitis C is a disease caused by viral infection with HCV, an RNA virus in the Flaviviridae family that predominately attacks the liver. In a small portion of acute cases, the body can eliminate the virus; however, the majority of acute cases develop into chronic infections. Chronic infections cause liver damage and may result in end-stage liver disease, or cirrhosis. Few of those persons who are chronically infected experience symptoms, and only one-third of acute cases develop jaundice or other symptoms. Chronic symptoms are nonspecific, intermittent, and mild, with the most common symptom being fatigue. Common symptoms of severe and advanced disease stages include nausea, dark urine, and jaundice. Since HCV infections are often asymptomatic, diagnosis

135

usually requires laboratory testing for both hepatitis antibodies (anti-HCV) which, when positive, indicate past or current infection, and the HCV nucleic acid (HCV RNA) which, when positive, indicates current infection. No vaccine protects against HCV infection, but new treatments have been reported to clear the infection and prevent advanced liver disease. [133,134,135]

Compared with other countries in the North Africa and Middle East region, Egypt has a high prevalence of HCV infection in the general population. In an attempt to treat endemic schistosomiasis, a condition caused by a common parasitic worm that affects the urinary tract, gut, and liver, the Egyptian Ministry of Health launched widespread injection-based treatment from 1950 to 1980. While there were improvements in schistosomiasis-induced mortality, recycled needles and poor needle sterilization used in delivering these medicines inadvertently infected many with HCV. [136,137,138] The spatial variations of HCV infection in North Africa and the Middle East provide a striking example for hierarchical random-effects modeling.

Random-effects modeling detects systematic differences among different spatial units of data. The spatial hierarchy in the GBD 2010 study uses countries nested in regions nested in superregions. There are 21 regions defined by demographic and epidemiological similarities, which are further clustered into seven superregions (see Appendix).

The analysis of HCV infection uses data on the prevalence of persons who have antibodies to HCV (anti-HCV). Incomplete data or data from high-risk populations, such as injection drug users or paid blood donors, were excluded. Figure 13.1 shows data collected in systematic review for two countries in the North Africa and Middle East region, Egypt and Jordan. Notice that for some age groups, anti-HCV prevalence measurements in Egypt are more than 40 times higher than the corresponding measurements in Jordan.

We used the age-standardizing, generalized negative-binomial spline model with hierarchical random effects to estimate anti-HCV prevalence. The hierarchical random effects allow the model to capture variation within the North Africa and Middle East region. Table 13.1 shows that Egypt has significantly higher prevalence than the other countries in the region. Figure 13.2 confirms this, as the prevalence estimate for Egypt is much above the regional average.

In addition to hierarchical random effects, the negative-binomial rate model included a parameter that estimates the amount of nonsampling error, parametrized as the overdispersion term δ (which can be interpreted as an observation-level random effect, as described in Chapter 2). In noisy data like this HCV seroprevalence dataset, priors on δ help with convergence and inform the pos-

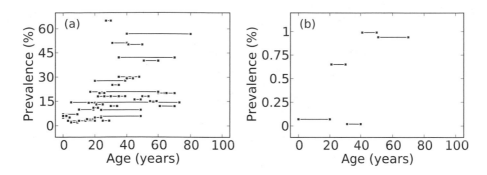

Figure 13.1. Prevalence data from systematic review of anti-HCV in (a) Egypt and (b) Jordan.

Table 13.1. Estimates of the country-level random effects for anti-HCV prevalence (an intercept shift in log-space) from the random-effects model for the countries in the North Africa and Middle East region.

Country	Posterior Mean	Lower 95% HPD	Upper 95% HPD
Egypt	1.87	1.5	2.2
Jordan	−0.59	−1.1	−0.1
Saudi Arabia	−0.77	−1.2	−0.4
Iraq	0.07	−0.4	0.6
Iran	0.02	−0.4	0.5
Yemen	0.04	−0.4	0.4
Turkey	−0.31	−0.7	0.0
Syria	−0.13	−0.7	0.4
Tunisia	−0.19	−0.7	0.3

terior estimates about beliefs regarding data heterogeneity. This allows the model to incorporate expert beliefs about how much of the country-to-country variation is true variation and how much is nonsampling error. We compared three alternative priors on the negative-binomial model dispersion parameter δ, corresponding to "very," "moderately," or "slightly" overdispersed. The natural logarithm of δ is uniformly distributed between its lower and upper bounds.

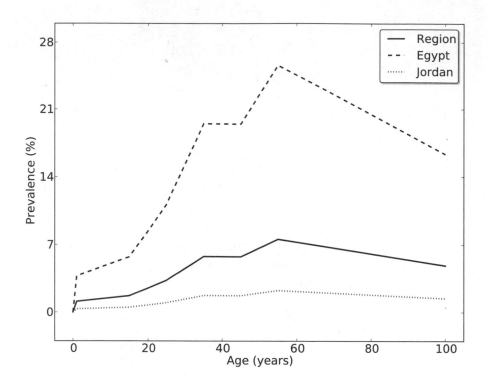

Figure 13.2. The 1990 estimate of anti-HCV prevalence for men in the North Africa and Middle East region and in the countries Egypt and Jordan. These estimates use only two levels in the hierarchical random-effects model: region and country.

Intended as a diffuse prior, the bounds of the categories of δ overlap, so that the bounds of "very," "moderately," and "slightly" are $[1, 9]$, $[3, 27]$, and $[9, 81]$, respectively.

In this example, the effects of priors on the overdispersion of δ are seen in the posterior estimates at the country level, as shown in Figure 13.3. The model is faced with the challenge of separating variation out into sampling error, nonsampling error between measurements (from a variety of indistinguishable causes, such as different study designs, different laboratory quality, or different response rates), and true variation between different populations.

With the amount of data available for fitting this model, a change in the prior on heterogeneity changes the posterior distribution of the level of variation noticeably, and thus also changes the estimated sizes of the random effects. As seen in Figure 13.3, when the prior on overdispersion is "very," the estimates are more compressed than those with a prior of "slightly."

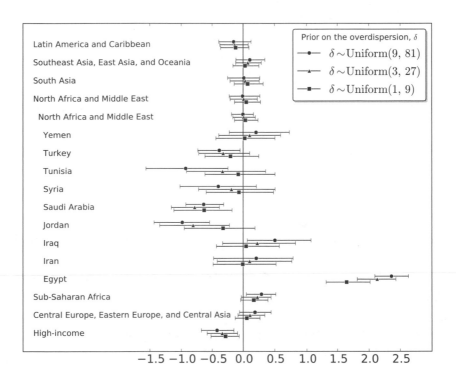

Figure 13.3. The intercept shift of anti-HCV prevalence for men in 1990 in log-space with different priors on global heterogeneity, δ. Four levels (global, superregion, region, country) were used in the hierarchical random-effects spline model in GBD 2010.

Another way to view compressed estimates is by looking at the age-standardized prevalence in Table 13.2. As heterogeneity increases from "slightly" to "very," country estimates are compressed toward the regional mean.

Hierarchical random effects and the overdispersion parameter δ allow the model to distinguish between true country-to-country variation and nonsam-

Table 13.2. Anti-HCV age-standardized prevalence estimates from a hierarchical random-effects spline model with differing priors on global heterogeneity.

Geographic Area	Heterogeneity	Posterior Mean	Standard Deviation
North Africa and Middle East	$\delta \sim \text{Uniform}(9, 81)$	0.048	0.003
	$\delta \sim \text{Uniform}(3, 27)$	0.049	0.004
	$\delta \sim \text{Uniform}(1, 9)$	0.045	0.005
Jordan	$\delta \sim \text{Uniform}(9, 81)$	0.007	0.002
	$\delta \sim \text{Uniform}(3, 27)$	0.010	0.003
	$\delta \sim \text{Uniform}(1, 9)$	0.020	0.007
Egypt	$\delta \sim \text{Uniform}(9, 81)$	0.188	0.012
	$\delta \sim \text{Uniform}(3, 27)$	0.179	0.018
	$\delta \sim \text{Uniform}(1, 9)$	0.137	0.019

pling error. Weakly informative priors on δ incorporate the modeler's beliefs about data heterogeneity, while the hierarchical random effects provide a way to model regional variation. When a predictive covariate is available, it generally should be used instead of (or in addition to) random effects to explain the country-to-country variation (as Chapter 15 will demonstrate), but in the absence of this, geographic random effects provide a mechanism to model the level of unexplained but true variation between different areas.

Chapter 14

Cross-walking with fixed effects: anxiety disorders

Amanda Baxter, Jed Blore, Abraham D. Flaxman, Theo Vos, and Harvey Whiteford

The data collected in systematic reviews often contain a variety of study types or diagnostic criteria, which create systematic biases in the data. An extreme example was found in the systematic review of diabetes prevalence, where there were 18 variants of diagnostic criteria. The systematic review of anxiety disorders provides a simpler example, which is the focus of this chapter. This systematic review collected studies that used a handful of different recall periods to ask about the presence of the disorders. The quantity of interest for estimation was point prevalence, the proportion of the population with the condition at an instant in time. We used a fixed-effect model to adjust for the bias introduced by studies that measured period (e.g., past-year) prevalence, since these studies also provide valuable information on the descriptive epidemiology of the condition. This bias adjustment by fixed-effect modeling is also called a "cross-walk."

Anxiety disorders include at least eight separate conditions, each characterized by prominent anxiety at a level that interferes with daily life. Not all anxiety disorders manifest in similar ways. While generalized anxiety disorder is typically marked by persistent worry, panic disorder is usually characterized by intense fear for discrete periods of time.[119] As much comorbidity exists between individual anxiety disorders, anxiety disorders were modeled together as a single condition in GBD 2010.

Anxiety disorders do not have a consistent recall period for the measurement of epidemiological rates. Therefore, the data from systematic review include studies with measurements of point prevalence and period prevalence (i.e., 6-month or past-year prevalence). The analysis excludes lifetime prevalence measurements because such estimates are particularly prone to recall bias. Due to the nonnegligible remission rate for anxiety disorders, period prevalence is typically higher than point prevalence, as seen in Figure 14.1.

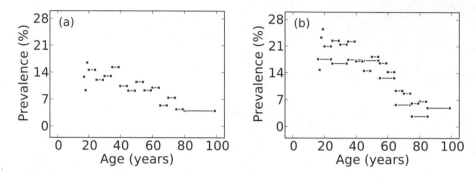

Figure 14.1. A comparison of (a) point and (b) period prevalence data for anxiety disorders in Australasian females, collected in a systematic review for 2000–2008.

Excluding period prevalence measurements reduces the quantity of data and produces results that do not reflect the regional variation present in the excluded data. But including the period prevalence measurements without a covariate to adjust for their systematic bias leads to estimates that are noticeably higher in regions where there are data on point and period prevalence. Using a fixed effect on a period prevalence indicator covariate allows the model to use all available data and explain the systematic bias and variation that result from different recall periods, as seen in Figure 14.2.

The results of the model with a fixed effect on recall period show that studies on period prevalence typically measure prevalence levels that are 49% (95% UI: [12, 91]) higher than if they measured point prevalence.

A limitation of applying this method to the global dataset is that it assumes the cross-walk factor is identical over age and sex for all regions of the world. This can be addressed by different cross-walks for different ages and sexes. In practice, there are rarely enough data to move beyond this assumption. However, future applications may benefit from random effects or modeling interactions between cross-walk covariates and age, sex, time, or geography.

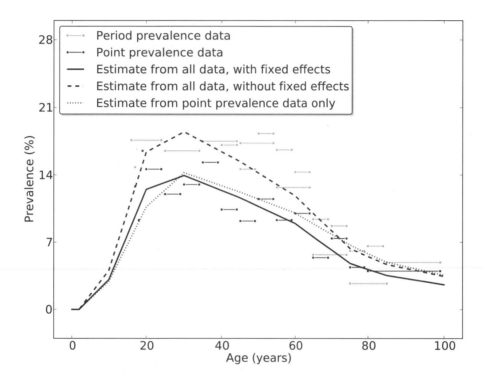

Figure 14.2. Comparison of prevalence estimates for anxiety disorders in 2005 in Australasian females using point prevalence data only, and using point and period prevalence data with and without a fixed effect.

Chapter 15

Improving out-of-sample prediction: liver cirrhosis

Ali Mokdad, Abraham D. Flaxman, Hannah M. Peterson,
Christopher J.L. Murray, and Mohsen Naghavi

Besides explaining the bias of noisy measurements as discussed in Chapter 14, fixed effects can also increase the accuracy of out-of-sample predictions. By modeling the relationship between the epidemiological parameter of interest and an explanatory covariate, the model can extrapolate estimates for areas where no direct measurements are available, using the inferred relationship with the known covariate data. For example, only a few regions have direct measurements for the prevalence of cirrhosis of the liver. However, by using the natural log of the age-standardized cirrhosis death rate as a country-level covariate to predict out-of-sample, it is possible to estimate the prevalence of cirrhosis in regions where there has been no direct measurement. Unlike the random-effects approach in Chapter 13, this approach attempts to explain the levels of national variation in this disease and not only capture their magnitude.

Cirrhosis of the liver is the result of chronic liver damage and is characterized by an advanced stage of liver fibrosis. Cirrhosis is the end stage of any chronic liver disease, with the most common causes being alcoholic liver disease and hepatitis B and C infections. Asymptomatic until a late stage of the disease, "compensated cirrhosis" may go undetected until complications develop. The diagnostic gold standard for cirrhosis is a liver biopsy. Complications such as jaundice, ascites, esophageal varices, and liver failure mark the progression from compensated to decompensated cirrhosis. The damage is irreversible, and cirrhosis management involves the prevention, control, and treatment of cirrhosis complications, with liver transplantation being the ultimate treatment. Without a liver transplant, mortality from decompensated cirrhosis is very high.[139,140,141]

Hospital databases yielded prevalence and cause-specific mortality rate data from four (of 21 possible) regions (Figure 15.1). Given the difficulty in cirrhosis diagnosis, it is assumed that these data represent decompensated cirrhosis, and the following analysis focuses on the symptomatic, decompensated phase of the disease.

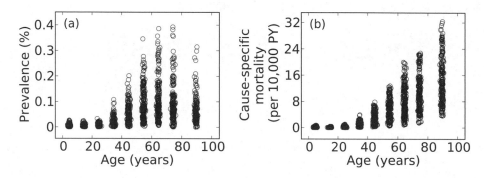

Figure 15.1. Available global data for cirrhosis (a) prevalence and (b) cause-specific mortality.

Since decompensated cirrhosis is a very severe condition, it is a sensible hypothesis that there is a strong association between prevalence and cause-specific mortality rate at the country level. In other words, we expected a priori that regions with higher death rates from cirrhosis would also have higher decompensated cirrhosis prevalence. Figure 15.2 shows the relationship between decompensated cirrhosis prevalence and the age-standardized death rate (ASDR) of cirrhosis as a scatterplot, using all data on cirrhosis prevalence collected in systematic review.

In regions with no cirrhosis data, estimates of the ASDR may be used as an explanatory covariate to estimate cirrhosis prevalence. By borrowing strength from the mortality estimates to inform the incidence estimates, cirrhosis prevalence can be estimated for regions without data, as shown in Figure 15.3. Since the predictive covariate fixed effects are modeled as a shift in log-space, it is often preferable to use the log of the ASDR as a covariate instead of using the ASDR untransformed.

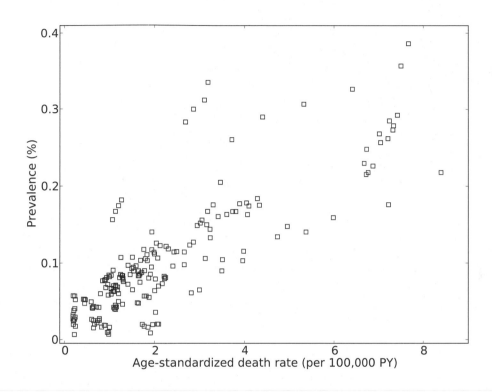

Figure 15.2. Relationship between cirrhosis prevalence data collected in systematic review and age-standardized death rate of cirrhosis.

As shown in Figure 15.3(b), despite the absence of any direct measurements of cirrhosis prevalence in Egypt, this approach provides a sensible estimate. It shows that the prevalence is much higher there than in the US. It also shows a sizable uncertainty interval, reflecting the imperfect relationship between prevalence and the ASDR. The age pattern is informed by borrowing strength from regions like North America where age-specific data are available.

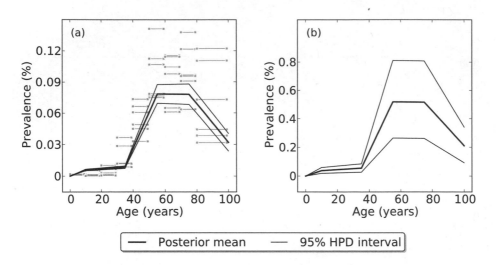

Figure 15.3. Cirrhosis prevalence estimates and available data for (a) the US and (b) Egypt, for males in 2005. Note that systematic review found no measurements of cirrhosis prevalence for Egypt, and prevalence level is extrapolated based on the inferred relationship with the age-standardized death rate.

Even in settings where there is not such a strong explanatory relationship between the parameter of interest and some covariate, this approach can still be useful. Although it would be ideal to have direct measurements of the quantities of interest, in many cases they have never been made. Explaining regional variation with a weak covariate is preferable to not explaining it at all.

Chapter 16

Risk factors: fruit consumption

Stephen S. Lim, Hannah M. Peterson,
and Abraham D. Flaxman

Although the primary focus of the metaregression framework developed in this book is on estimating prevalence of disease, it is also useful for estimating other age-specific quantities of interest in descriptive epidemiology. Subsequent chapters will address the consistent estimation framework that allows data on incidence, remission, and mortality to be included in estimates of prevalence; this approach produces estimates of age-specific incidence, remission, and mortality as ancillary outputs. But before turning to that, this chapter considers the possibility of using the age-standardizing mixed-effects spline model to produce estimates of risk factor exposures.

An important component of GBD 2010 was the estimation of disease burden attributable to risk factors, such as the lack of fresh fruit. Fruit consumption is a nonnegative quantity, so it is acceptable to model it with the negative-binomial rate model. This is somewhat inelegant, however, because this model assumes that the underlying quantity being measured is count data. A count model is appropriate for prevalence and incidence rates, which represent, for example, how many cases were observed during a certain period of observation. However, a continuous distribution, such as one of the transformed normal models from Chapter 2, is more common for modeling a quantity like kilograms of fruit consumed per day per capita. In this chapter, we will compare the results of using the negative-binomial rate model with two more traditional models for continuous data: the normal model and the lognormal model.

Fruit consumption has a significant protective effect against morbidity and mortality from several diseases. Measured as the total intake of fruit per day (kg/d), fruit includes all fresh, frozen, cooked, canned, or dried fruits, excluding fruit juices and salted or pickled fruits.[142,143]

Systematic reviews for risk factor epidemiology proceed much the same as for disease prevalence, at least for determining the population-level exposure to the risk. In the case of lack of fruit, systematic review collected 1,502 data points on age-specific consumption of fruit.

As discussed above, the negative binomial, normal, and lognormal models differ in their treatment of numbers that are very close to zero, but, with well-behaved data, the model estimates are largely independent of the choice of rate model, as seen in Figure 16.1, which compares estimates for models fitted to data from the US in 2005.

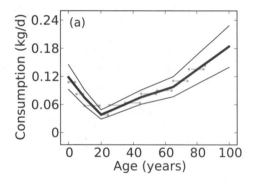 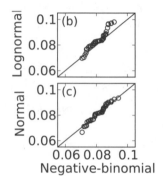

Figure 16.1. Estimates of fruit consumption in males in the US in 2005. (a) shows age-specific estimate using negative binomial model, (b) and (c) compare the posterior distribution of age-standardized consumption estimate of the negative-binomial model to the estimates using the lognormal and normal rate models.

In a setting where the data are sparser and noisier, the models still yield quite similar results, as shown in Figure 16.2 for data from Western Europe in 2005. It is worth noting that unlike the estimates in Figure 16.1, Figure 16.2 estimates do not go through the data at the youngest ages (0 to 20 years). This is because fruit consumption has substantial country-level random effects, shown with a comparison of Iceland and Greece in Figure 16.3.

In Figure 16.3, small differences in the estimates at the country level are noticeable. Table 16.1 shows that the mean age-standardized country estimates differ by rate type. However, while estimates at the country level differ slightly, the regional estimate remains the same.

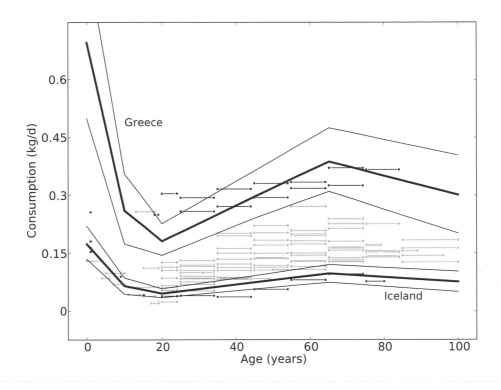

Figure 16.2. Fruit consumption estimates in Greece and Iceland for males in 2005 using the negative-binomial rate models.

The country-level estimate for Greece also highlights a challenge for this approach. Since there are no data from Greece for the youngest age groups, the model borrows strength from other countries in the region. But since these countries are lower than average in adult consumption, while Greece is higher, the model predicts very high consumption in children. Assuming the same relationship in country-to-country variation for children as for adults seems reasonable in theory, and indeed there are no data to contradict this; however, the resulting estimates are substantially above any of the levels measured in the region. This is suspicious and certainly justifies additional investigation.

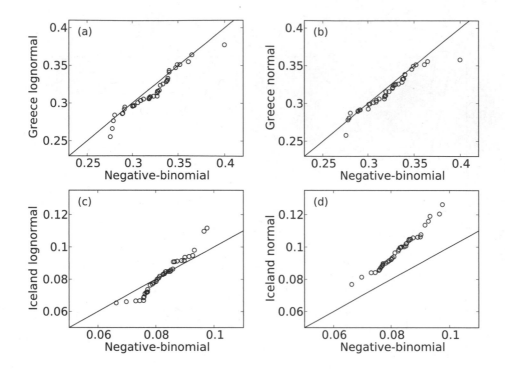

Figure 16.3. Comparison of posterior distribution of age-standardized fruit consumption estimates using different rate models in Greece in 2005: using the negative-binomial model and (a) the lognormal rate model (b) the normal rate model; and in Iceland in 2005: using the negative-binomial model and (c) the lognormal rate model and (d) the normal rate model.

It could also call for incorporating additional priors into the model, based on expert knowledge about the absolute levels, country-to-country variation, or smoothness or monotonicity of the age pattern.

On the topic of country-to-country variation, this model is also a good example for how future work might go beyond the countries-nested-in-regions-nested-in-superregions hierarchical approach to borrowing strength. It is reasonable to hypothesize that the fruit consumption in Greece and Italy is more similar than in Greece and Ireland, and in general, that countries within Western Europe that are closer together will have more similar exposures to nutritional risk factors. This could be represented in the model, using the conditionally autoregressive approach of spatial statistics, for example.[144]

Table 16.1. Random-effect estimates from hierarchical spline models of fruit consumption with differing rate models.

Model	Iceland	[95% UI]	Greece	[95% UI]
Negative-binomial	-0.57	$[-0.8, -0.4]$	0.81	$[0.7, 1.0]$
Lognormal	-0.55	$[-0.7, -0.4]$	0.80	$[0.6, 1.0]$
Normal	-0.41	$[-0.6, -0.2]$	0.78	$[0.7, 0.9]$

With ample data, different rate models produce small differences in moderately noisy data, mostly at the country level. Similar estimates from the negative-binomial, normal, and lognormal rate models only build confidence that the model is not sensitive to the choice of these rate types. When the data are sparser or noisier, considering the difference between estimates produced by different models can be a useful component of a sensitivity analysis.

Chapter 17

The compartmental model: end-stage renal disease

Sarah K. Wulf, Abraham D. Flaxman, Mohsen Naghavi, and Giuseppe Remuzzi

We now turn our attention to conditions where systematic review uncovered a substantial amount of epidemiological data on incidence, remission, and mortality, which we wish to use to inform our estimates of prevalence. This was already touched on in Chapter 12 and will be investigated more systematically in the next few chapters. We begin by considering end-stage renal disease (ESRD) treated with dialysis, a condition for which data on prevalence, incidence, remission, and with-condition mortality were all collected in relatively large quantities through systematic review.

ESRD is the final stage of chronic kidney disease (CKD), the slow and progressive loss of kidney function. The most common causes of CKD are diabetes and high blood pressure. Damage to kidneys is usually permanent, but treatment and lifestyle changes can slow disease progression. However, at the final stage of the disease, the kidneys no longer function, and the patient needs dialysis or a kidney transplant to survive. There are two main types of dialysis for kidney treatment: hemodialysis and peritoneal dialysis. Hemodialysis filters waste and excess fluids from the blood externally using a machine, while peritoneal dialysis uses the lining of the peritoneal cavity and a catheter to filter wastes from the blood. [145,146]

This example focuses on ESRD treated with dialysis, combining hemodialysis and peritoneal dialysis for analysis. Most of the data are from studies or registry reports. Transplantation incidence among the prevalent dialysis population was used as a proxy for remission. The analysis includes 5,664 data points representing 161 countries in all 21 GBD 2010 regions. Data from Australasia are shown in Figure 17.1.

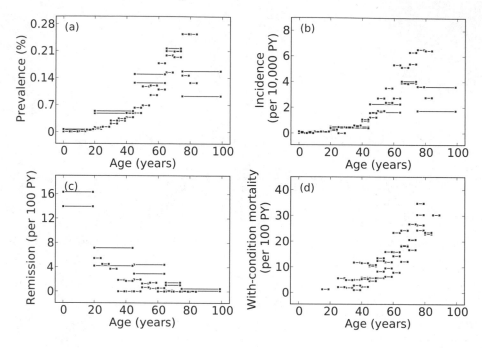

Figure 17.1. Four types of data for Australasian males with ESRD treated with dialysis in 2005: (a) prevalence, (b) incidence, (c) remission, and (d) with-condition mortality.

As discussed in Section 7.2, epidemiological parameters, such as incidence, prevalence, remission, and with-condition mortality, are related by a logical requirement of internal consistency. A prevalent case can exist only if there was a past incident event, and the current number of prevalent cases can be determined from past prevalent cases, newly incident cases, deaths, and remissions. Modeling the parameters simultaneously produces a best estimate and plausible uncertainty bounds for incidence and prevalence that are internally consistent for a single time, place, and sex.

Figure 17.2 compares the compartmental and spline model results for Australasian males with ESRD treated with dialysis in 2005. While the spline model estimates each epidemiological parameter individually, the compartmental model estimates prevalence, incidence, remission, and with-condition mortality simultaneously. Figure 17.2 and a comparison of the age-standardized prevalence estimates for the region show that the compartmental model estimates do not follow the data like the spline model does. As seen in Figure 17.3, the spline model produces prevalence estimates that are systematically lower than those of the compartmental model because of the logic requirement that all prevalent cases have a corresponding incident event.

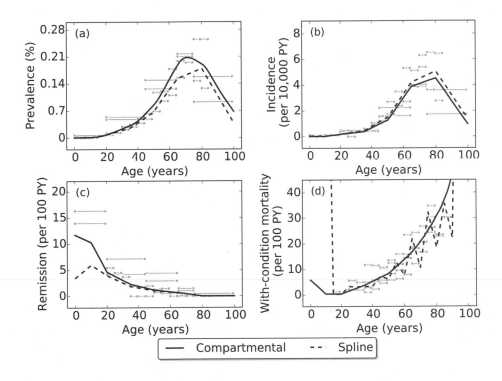

Figure 17.2. Comparison of epidemiological parameter estimates for Australasian males with ESRD treated with dialysis in 2005 using the compartmental and spline models.

Another advantage to compartmental modeling is an estimate with a smooth age pattern. Modeling each epidemiological parameter individually, the spline model follows the data exactly, often producing an uneven age pattern, as seen in Figure 17.4. This effect can be minimized by placing an informative prior on the penalized spline model as discussed in Chapter 3.

The compartmental model is preferable to modeling each parameter individually with the spline model because it incorporates all available data.

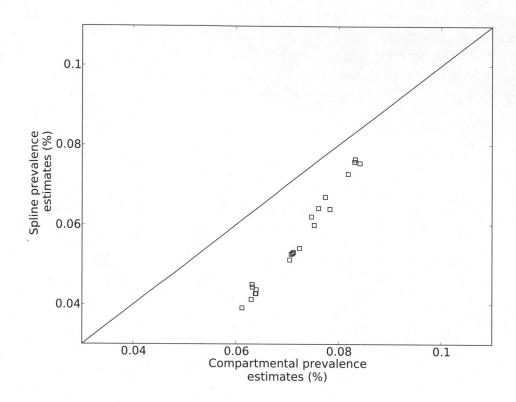

Figure 17.3. Comparison of the regional age-standardized prevalence estimates using compartmental and spline models for males with ESRD treated with dialysis in 2005.

Simultaneously modeling all data, the compartmental model produces internally consistent estimates for a single age, sex, and time.

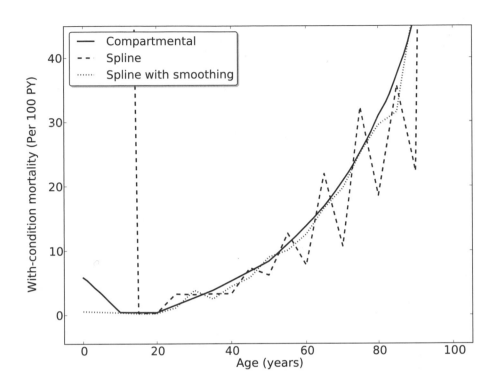

Figure 17.4. With-condition mortality estimates for Australasian males with ESRD treated with dialysis in 2005, using a compartmental model, a spline model, and a spline model with a smoothing parameter.

Chapter 18

Knot selection in compartmental spline models: osteoarthritis of the knee

Marita Cross, Damian Hoy, Theo Vos, Abraham D. Flaxman, and Lyn March

Chapters 9 and 10 demonstrated the importance of knot selection in spline models for sparse, noisy data. In this chapter, we return to this point in the context of compartmental models where the age-specific hazards are represented by splines, and the parameter of primary interest, prevalence, comes from the solution to a system of differential equations based on these splines. In this setting, modeling decisions about the knot locations for one parameter affect the estimates for all the other parameters. The compartmental model for osteoarthritis of the knee provides a demonstration of this.

Osteoarthritis (OA) is a disorder that affects joint cartilage and underlying bone. OA causes pain in the joints and limits movement. OA of the knee is common and causes significant morbidity, particularly in the elderly.[147,148] Systematic review yielded 602 data points representing 27 countries in 10 GBD 2010 regions.

Since OA of the knee is exceedingly rare in young adults, expert priors inform the model that the onset of the disease does not start before age 30. The number and location of knots in the incidence rate after this minimum age of onset determine critical features of the model. As shown in Figure 18.1, it is important to have enough knots to represent the rapid change in age-specific incidence. However, knot selection in incidence also affects estimates of prevalence and excess mortality.

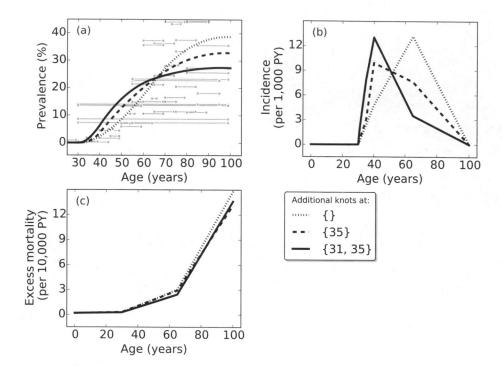

Figure 18.1. Knot selection between the ages of 30 and 99 plays an important role in the estimates of (a) prevalence, (b) incidence, and (c) excess mortality for Western European females with OA of the knee in 2005. The incidence rate of all models has knots at $\{0, 30, 40, 45, 65, 100\}$. Between the ages of 30 and 40, the models have either no additional knots ($\{\}$) or additional knots at $\{35\}$ or $\{31, 35\}$.

The model is also sensitive to assumptions about the epidemiological profile, expressed in the model as expert priors. Figure 18.2 compares assumptions about incidence of OA of the knee. A prior that requires zero incidence at ages greater than 99 implies that incidence decreases with age. In other words, after a certain age, if OA of the knee has not developed, it is unlikely it ever will. Without this prior, incidence increases with age. The logic requirement of internal consistency in the compartmental model means that prevalence estimates are also affected, as shown in Figure 18.2. When incidence is unrestricted, prevalence has a very different age pattern than when incidence is restricted.

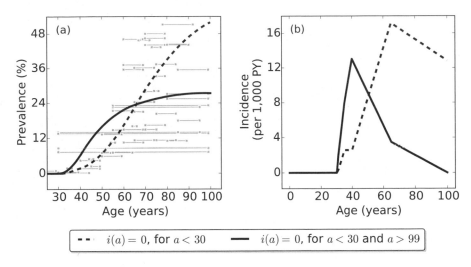

Figure 18.2. A comparison of (a) prevalence and (b) incidence estimates for Western European females with OA of the knee in 2005, with and without a prior stipulating no onset of the disease in ages greater than 99 using a compartmental model.

Knot selection had a substantial effect on the estimates, although it can be minimized by increasing the number of knots included in the model. Likewise, informative priors on incidence drastically modified other parameter estimates. With ample data, the consistent model is robust to knot selection. When there are not enough data, knot selection should be based on principled considerations and a sensitivity analysis performed. The sensitivity analysis shows the effect of assumptions and the range of results, allowing the modeler to understand the differences arising from different assumptions. The influence of priors in compartmental modeling is elaborated further in the following chapter.

Chapter 19

Expert priors in compartmental models: bipolar disorder

Alizé Ferrari, Abraham D. Flaxman, Hannah M. Peterson,
Theo Vos, and Harvey Whiteford

Just as priors in the spline model were influential on the estimates produced for PMS prevalence in Chapter 10, the priors on the age-specific rates in a compartmental model can be influential on the estimates. The situation is more complicated here, however, because priors on a hazard of one type propagate through to affect the estimates for all other parameters as well, due to the consistency enforced by the compartmental model. In this chapter, we will use the meta-analysis of bipolar disorder prevalence as an example of the effects of informative priors on levels of age-specific incidence and remission hazards.

Bipolar disorder is a mental disorder that causes the experience of at least one manic and one major depressive episode, interspersed by periods of residual symptoms. A manic episode is characterized by elevated, expansive, or irritable mood, while a depressive episode is characterized by depressed mood or loss of interest in everyday activities. A shift between episodes is demarcated by either a change in symptoms to the opposite polarity or experiences of residual symptoms that are below the threshold for a manic or depressive episode. In the case of rapid cycling, shifts between episodes occur as frequently as four or more shifts in a given year. Extreme behavior changes accompany mood changes, and it is not uncommon for sleeping, eating, or activity patterns to change with manic and depressive episodes. While there is no cure, treatment helps manage mood swings and related symptoms.[149,150]

The modeling of bipolar disorder is based on literature describing it as a chronic illness with little or no complete remission. The terms "residual" and "remission" have very different implications for GBD 2010. A residual state involves less severe symptoms with lesser disability but still contributes to disease burden. Remission is equivalent to a cure rather than a temporary reduction in symptom levels and thus does not contribute to burden. No studies were found reporting on complete remission from bipolar disorder as per this definition, which is consistent with the description in the literature that there is no cure.[119] In this chapter, analysis uses only data from high-income North America, as shown in Figure 19.1.

While some evidence suggests that bipolar disorder commonly starts in the midteens or early twenties, there is still disagreement over a minimum age of onset. Even though symptoms can be tracked back to childhood, setting a

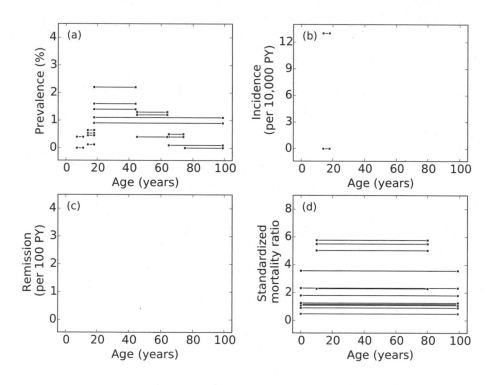

Figure 19.1. Data on (a) prevalence, (b) incidence, (c) remission, and (d) standardized mortality ratio collected from systematic review of bipolar disorder in high-income North America.

threshold for diagnosis is difficult, given that current diagnostic criteria are based on the adult presentation of the disorder. Literature and expert advice suggest that although prepubertal bipolar disorder is rare, it may possibly exist. [149,150]

While expert priors are useful in guiding the modeling process, they may have unintended effects, as discussed in Chapter 4. Choosing to have no restrictions on the age of onset alters the age-specific prevalence greatly, as shown in Figure 19.2.

Like the age of onset, little is known about the upper age limit of incidence of bipolar disorder. Using expert knowledge to set plausible bounds on the

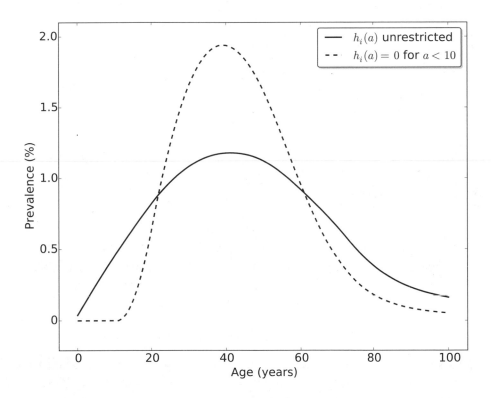

Figure 19.2. Estimates of the prevalence of bipolar disorder for males in the GBD 2010 region of high-income North America in 1990 using differing priors for age of onset in a compartmental model.

level of disease is useful in modeling noisy data. However, changes in the upper age limit may produce unexpected changes, as shown in Figure 19.3. The prevalence estimates in Figure 19.3 are about the same because there are enough data to inform the model, but incidence, remission, and excess mortality undergo subtle changes to account for the prior.

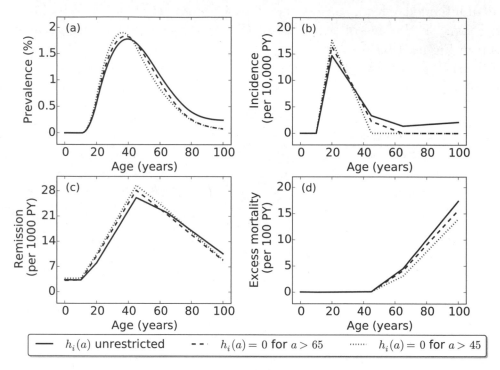

Figure 19.3. Estimated (a) prevalence, (b) incidence, (c) remission, and (d) excess mortality for males with bipolar disorder in the GBD 2010 region of high-income North America in 1990, using a compartmental model with different priors on the upper age limit of incidence of 45 years, 65 years, or unrestricted.

In sparse and noisy data, sometimes the changes to account for the prior are not so subtle, as shown in the sensitivity analysis in Figure 19.4. Here, small changes in the prior level on remission lead to large changes in the estimated excess mortality.

The internal consistency in the compartmental model causes modeling decisions, such as priors on level, for one parameter to propagate and affect all other parameter estimates. When working with ample data, the model esti-

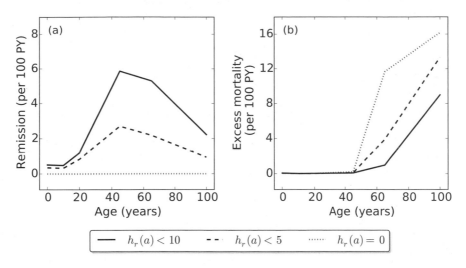

Figure 19.4. Estimated (a) remission and (b) excess mortality for bipolar disorder in males in high-income North America in 1990, in a compartmental model with different priors on remission that limit remission to 0, 5, or 10 per 100 PY.

mates are robust against the choice of informative priors on level. However, these choices can cause substantial changes to estimates when working with sparse and noisy data.

Chapter 20

Cause-specific mortality rates: alcohol dependence

Theo Vos, Jed Blore, Abraham D. Flaxman,
Hannah M. Peterson, and Juergen Rehm

A key assumption of the years of life lost (YLL) estimates in GBD 2010 is that only one cause leads to death. This categorical attribution of deaths in a mutually exclusive way has the desirable property that all assigned deaths sum to the total number of deaths. However, this creates a rate that does not directly correspond to any rate in the compartmental model (Figure 7.3). Using this cause-specific mortality rate (CSMR) as a measurement of $p \cdot h_f$ forces the assumption that all who die *with* the condition die *of* the condition. While this is a reasonable assumption for conditions such as cancer, cirrhosis, or diarrhea, it is not for conditions such as alcohol dependence, where many people die *with* the condition but *not of* it. Using alcohol dependence as an example, this chapter compares the results of the modeling assumptions of those who die *of* alcohol dependence and those who die *with* alcohol dependence but of other causes.

Alcohol dependence is the dysfunctional pattern of alcohol consumption that leads to physiological dependence and impaired control. Similar to cocaine dependence (Chapter 9), in order to be diagnosed with alcohol dependence, three or more of the seven substance dependence criteria identified by the American Psychiatric Association must be fulfilled within a 12-month period.[119,151] Systematic review yielded prevalence, excess mortality, and cause-specific mortality data as seen in Figure 20.1.

To include cause-specific mortality data in the compartmental model, the model in Figure 7.3 can be adapted by splitting the excess mortality h_f into

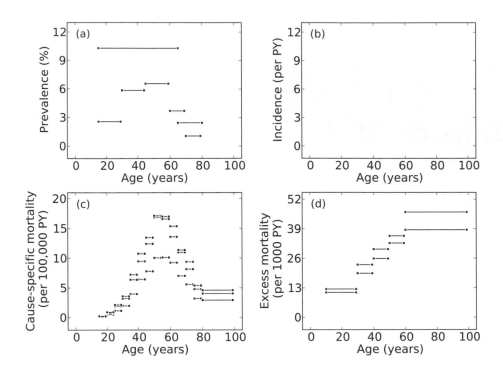

Figure 20.1. Data on alcohol dependence in males from the GBD 2010 region of Central Asia, collected by systematic review for (a) prevalence, (b) incidence, (c) cause-specific mortality, and (d) excess mortality.

two parts (Figure 20.2): those who die *of* the condition $h_{f'}$ and those who die *with* the condition but *not of* it $h_{f''}$. As described in Section 2.7, excess mortality can then be represented as

$$h_f = h_{f''} + h_{f'}$$

While the product of excess mortality and prevalence, $p \cdot h_f$, can be directly measured, in practice $h_{f''}$ and $h_{f'}$ are never disentangled. Our method implicitly separates $h_{f'}$ and $h_{f''}$ but does not try to explicitly represent both.

For some diseases in GBD 2010, it is a reasonable assumption that $h_{f''} = 0$, so that those who die with the condition die of it. When this is the case, the cause-specific mortality is a direct estimate of $p \cdot h_f$, a measurement of population mortality. However, for diseases such as alcohol dependence, this

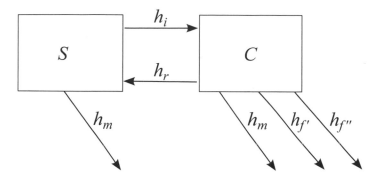

Figure 20.2. The two-compartment mechanistic model with the excess mortality split into two hazards.

is a questionable assumption, for the reasons mentioned above. When $h_{f''} \neq 0$, cause-specific mortality data provide the lower bound on $p \cdot h_f$.

As seen in Figure 20.3, assuming $h_{f''} = 0$ instead of $h_{f''} \geq 0$ leads to a change in the estimated prevalence of the condition.

By decomposing excess mortality into those who die of the disease and those who die with the disease but not of the disease, the compartmental model in Figure 7.3 can use the cause-specific mortality data as a lower bound on prevalence times excess mortality, which is appropriate if the disease is not exclusively coded as the underlying cause of death.

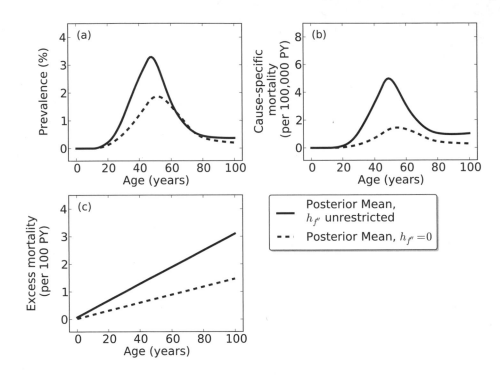

Figure 20.3. Comparison of (a) prevalence, (b) cause-specific mortality, and (c) excess mortality estimates of alcohol dependence in Central Asian males in 2005, when using cause-specific mortality data as a lower bound ($h_{f''}$ unrestricted) or a direct estimate of the product of prevalence and excess mortality ($h_{f''} = 0$).

Conclusion

Abraham D. Flaxman, Christopher J.L. Murray,
and Theo Vos

This book has developed our new metaregression framework for descriptive epidemiology from first principles and applied it to several examples. This approach is complicated because the data have many complex features that must be addressed. However, we have addressed each of these complex features one by one, aiming to make it less imposing than having to consider the sum of the parts.

There are seven ways that this approach differs from traditional meta-analysis, each addressing commonly occurring features of the data collected in systematic review during GBD 2010. Recall that the data are often very *sparse* and very *noisy*; there are whole regions of the globe for which no data are available; at times there are no measurements of prevalence, but only of incidence; regions that do have data may have measurements that vary 10 times more than sampling error would allow; and in many combinations of these challenging environments, we must produce estimates that reflect the uncertainty of the available data.

Our approach has used the following:

- The negative binomial model of data, an approach that allows zero observations and dispersion beyond what can be accommodated in Poisson and binomial models.

- A piecewise linear spline model of age-specific hazards, which balances computational tractability and age-pattern flexibility.

- Bayesian methods, to quantify uncertainty and incorporate priors based on biology or clinical knowledge.

- The age-standardizing model of heterogeneous, nonstandard age groups, such as 18–35 or 15 and older.

- Fixed effects modeling to crosswalk between available studies that use different study methods; to predict out-of-sample, based on known country-specific covariates; and to quantify differences in nonsampling variance in different study types.

- Random effects modeling to capture true variation within and between regions.

- Integrative systems modeling to combine and make consistent data collected for many different outcomes, such as incidence, prevalence, remission, excess mortality, or cause-specific mortality.

These methods have extended traditional metaregression in a number of directions, but the field should and will continue to evolve. The comprehensive systematic reviews of published and unpublished data conducted for the GBD 2010 study constitute a wide variety of application areas. Unexpected findings in the descriptive epidemiology of these conditions should prompt additional data collection for confirmation, and should guide where new methods need to be developed.

There are a number of important extensions to this approach and other avenues for future work that should be pursued in the future. These have been highlighted at the end of each chapter in Part I of the book, and are collated here, as a plan for moving forward.

Now that systematic reviews have been conducted for numerous conditions, the data gathered in the reviews can be used for a systematic out-of-sample cross-validation, where some of the data are withheld and compared with the model predictions, to refine modeling choices and suggest new improvements.

Further research into the rate models from Chapter 2 can continue to develop and test the offset log-transformed model and see how it compares to the negative binomial model on a range of models collected through systematic review. Perhaps with additional innovation in computation algorithms, the beta-binomial model can also be made efficient enough to be seriously considered as well, but this seems to require methods beyond the MCMC approach of Chapter 8.

The age-specific hazard functions in Chapter 3 have more model parameters than would be ideal. Future work should be dedicated to removing the necessity of spline-modeling decisions about the number of knots, location of knots, and level of smoothing. If computational algorithms become fast enough, this could be accomplished simply by exploring a range of parameters and selecting (or averaging) based on cross-validation using out-of-sample predictive validity. An alternative line of research would be to go from spline models to Gaussian processes, or some related nonparametric formulation of age-specific hazard function. This will certainly have its own computational challenges.

The priors in Chapter 4 can be extended through three directions of future work. First, the expert priors deserve an automated and foolproof procedure for sensitivity analysis (perhaps based on out-of-sample cross validation, if it is computationally feasible), so the impact of these assumptions can be assessed quickly and comprehensively. Second, there are additional formulations of expert priors that would be helpful in certain settings, such as the unimodality prior described at the end of that chapter. Third, and most important, the empirical priors that have been used so far must be compared to alternative formulations, particularly in terms of the assumptions about the variance-covariance matrix for the joint distribution of hazards at different ages; a stark example of this is in modeling mild congenital conditions, where uncertainty in birth prevalence propagates through to all ages, and seeing a higher than average prevalence at age 10 should not be at all surprising to someone who saw a higher-than-average prevalence at age zero.

Age-group modeling and covariate modeling can be extended to consider alternative models of heterogeneous age groups, uncertainty, and missingness in predictive covariates. Based on the success of ensemble modeling for covariates in other settings, that approach could also be considered here, but only if the computation time for individual models in the ensemble can be sped up substantially first.

The countries-nested-in-regions-nested-in-superregions hierarchical approach to random effects is another area for particular attention. Instead of grouping areal units hierarchically, it could be fruitful to use a model that took the distance between areas (geographically or sociopolitically) more directly into account. The conditionally autoregressive models developed in the spatial statistics literature provide a specific direction to follow for this line of research.

Removing the endemic equilibrium assumption from Section 7.3 is another important direction for future work. The available data for most global descriptive epidemiology are too sparse and noisy to justify this complication, but for many national and subnational analyses, this will be highly relevant.

All these directions for future work will be facilitated by research into numerical algorithms and computational infrastructure, since the time it takes to run these models is currently an impediment to large cross-validation exercises, as well as searching for optimal parameter settings through out-of-sample predictive validity.

If substantial speed increases are possible through improved algorithms and infrastructure, it may also be possible to go beyond the empirical Bayes approach and to fit a full hierarchical model for all regions (or countries) simultaneously. This will require innovation in models as well as methods to determine the most appropriate way to formalize the hierarchical similarity priors. It is likely to be extremely demanding computationally, however, and experimenting with alternative approaches to the empirical prior model could yield an intermediate approach that requires only a more modest increase in computational power.

Besides computational algorithms and speed, another area of research is to create more tools for the analyst to compare different rate types and the effects of modeling decisions. In particular, developing an exploratory graphical method to determine the effect of the priors and the effect of the data on the posterior estimate would be valuable for model checking.

Any counterintuitive findings based on these methods should be interpreted with caution, especially in cases where the results have important policy implications. Our new metaregression model can tease estimates out of sparse and noisy data, but it is important to remember that these estimates often have substantial uncertainty.

The development of a metaregression approach for descriptive epidemiological prediction has been quite an adventure. It is likely to continue to be in the future as data, models, methods, and infrastructure change and improve, making even more precise and accurate estimation possible.

Appendix

GBD Study 2010 spatial hierarchy

Table A.1. Spatial hierarchy used in the GBD Study 2010

GBD superregion	GDB region	Country	ISO3
Central Europe, Eastern Europe, and Central Asia	Central Asia	Armenia	ARM
Central Europe, Eastern Europe, and Central Asia	Central Asia	Azerbaijan	AZE
Central Europe, Eastern Europe, and Central Asia	Central Asia	Georgia	GEO
Central Europe, Eastern Europe, and Central Asia	Central Asia	Kazakhstan	KAZ
Central Europe, Eastern Europe, and Central Asia	Central Asia	Kyrgyzstan	KGZ
Central Europe, Eastern Europe, and Central Asia	Central Asia	Mongolia	MNG
Central Europe, Eastern Europe, and Central Asia	Central Asia	Tajikistan	TJK
Central Europe, Eastern Europe, and Central Asia	Central Asia	Turkmenistan	TKM
Central Europe, Eastern Europe, and Central Asia	Central Asia	Uzbekistan	UZB

Table A.1. (continued)

GBD superregion	GDB region	Country	ISO3
Central Europe, Eastern Europe, and Central Asia	Central Europe	Albania	ALB
Central Europe, Eastern Europe, and Central Asia	Central Europe	Bosnia and Herzegovina	BIH
Central Europe, Eastern Europe, and Central Asia	Central Europe	Bulgaria	BGR
Central Europe, Eastern Europe, and Central Asia	Central Europe	Croatia	HRV
Central Europe, Eastern Europe, and Central Asia	Central Europe	Czech Republic	CZE
Central Europe, Eastern Europe, and Central Asia	Central Europe	Hungary	HUN
Central Europe, Eastern Europe, and Central Asia	Central Europe	Macedonia	MKD
Central Europe, Eastern Europe, and Central Asia	Central Europe	Montenegro	MNE
Central Europe, Eastern Europe, and Central Asia	Central Europe	Poland	POL
Central Europe, Eastern Europe, and Central Asia	Central Europe	Romania	ROU
Central Europe, Eastern Europe, and Central Asia	Central Europe	Serbia	SRB
Central Europe, Eastern Europe, and Central Asia	Central Europe	Slovakia	SVK
Central Europe, Eastern Europe, and Central Asia	Central Europe	Slovenia	SVN
Central Europe, Eastern Europe, and Central Asia	Eastern Europe	Belarus	BLR
Central Europe, Eastern Europe, and Central Asia	Eastern Europe	Estonia	EST
Central Europe, Eastern Europe, and Central Asia	Eastern Europe	Latvia	LVA
Central Europe, Eastern Europe, and Central Asia	Eastern Europe	Lithuania	LTU

Table A.1. (continued)

GBD superregion	GDB region	Country	ISO3
Central Europe, Eastern Europe, and Central Asia	Eastern Europe	Moldova	MDA
Central Europe, Eastern Europe, and Central Asia	Eastern Europe	Russia	RUS
Central Europe, Eastern Europe, and Central Asia	Eastern Europe	Ukraine	UKR
High-income	Australasia	Australia	AUS
High-income	Australasia	New Zealand	NZL
High-income	High-income Asia Pacific	Brunei	BRN
High-income	High-income Asia Pacific	Japan	JPN
High-income	High-income Asia Pacific	South Korea	KOR
High-income	High-income Asia Pacific	Singapore	SGP
High-income	High-income North America	Canada	CAN
High-income	High-income North America	USA	USA
High-income	Southern Latin America	Argentina	ARG
High-income	Southern Latin America	Chile	CHL
High-income	Southern Latin America	Uruguay	URY
High-income	Western Europe	Andorra	AND
High-income	Western Europe	Austria	AUT
High-income	Western Europe	Belgium	BEL
High-income	Western Europe	Cyprus	CYP
High-income	Western Europe	Denmark	DNK
High-income	Western Europe	Finland	FIN
High-income	Western Europe	France	FRA
High-income	Western Europe	Germany	DEU
High-income	Western Europe	Greece	GRC

Table A.1. (continued)

GBD superregion	GDB region	Country	ISO3
High-income	Western Europe	Iceland	ISL
High-income	Western Europe	Ireland	IRL
High-income	Western Europe	Israel	ISR
High-income	Western Europe	Italy	ITA
High-income	Western Europe	Luxembourg	LUX
High-income	Western Europe	Malta	MLT
High-income	Western Europe	Netherlands	NLD
High-income	Western Europe	Norway	NOR
High-income	Western Europe	Portugal	PRT
High-income	Western Europe	Spain	ESP
High-income	Western Europe	Sweden	SWE
High-income	Western Europe	Switzerland	CHE
High-income	Western Europe	UK	GBR
Latin America and Caribbean	Andean Latin America	Bolivia	BOL
Latin America and Caribbean	Andean Latin America	Ecuador	ECU
Latin America and Caribbean	Andean Latin America	Peru	PER
Latin America and Caribbean	Caribbean	Antigua and Barbuda	ATG
Latin America and Caribbean	Caribbean	Bahamas	BHS
Latin America and Caribbean	Caribbean	Barbados	BRB
Latin America and Caribbean	Caribbean	Belize	BLZ
Latin America and Caribbean	Caribbean	Bermuda	BMU
Latin America and Caribbean	Caribbean	Cuba	CUB
Latin America and Caribbean	Caribbean	Dominica	DMA
Latin America and Caribbean	Caribbean	Dominican Republic	DOM

Table A.1. (continued)

GBD superregion	GDB region	Country	ISO3
Latin America and Caribbean	Caribbean	Grenada	GRD
Latin America and Caribbean	Caribbean	Guyana	GUY
Latin America and Caribbean	Caribbean	Haiti	HTI
Latin America and Caribbean	Caribbean	Jamaica	JAM
Latin America and Caribbean	Caribbean	Puerto Rico	PRI
Latin America and Caribbean	Caribbean	Saint Lucia	LCA
Latin America and Caribbean	Caribbean	Saint Vincent and the Grenadines	VCT
Latin America and Caribbean	Caribbean	Suriname	SUR
Latin America and Caribbean	Caribbean	Trinidad and Tobago	TTO
Latin America and Caribbean	Central Latin America	Colombia	COL
Latin America and Caribbean	Central Latin America	Costa Rica	CRI
Latin America and Caribbean	Central Latin America	El Salvador	SLV
Latin America and Caribbean	Central Latin America	Guatemala	GTM
Latin America and Caribbean	Central Latin America	Honduras	HND
Latin America and Caribbean	Central Latin America	Mexico	MEX
Latin America and Caribbean	Central Latin America	Nicaragua	NIC
Latin America and Caribbean	Central Latin America	Panama	PAN

Table A.1. (continued)

GBD superregion	GDB region	Country	ISO3
Latin America and Caribbean	Central Latin America	Venezuela	VEN
Latin America and Caribbean	Tropical Latin America	Brazil	BRA
Latin America and Caribbean	Tropical Latin America	Paraguay	PRY
North Africa and Middle East	North Africa and Middle East	Afghanistan	AFG
North Africa and Middle East	North Africa and Middle East	Algeria	DZA
North Africa and Middle East	North Africa and Middle East	Bahrain	BHR
North Africa and Middle East	North Africa and Middle East	Egypt	EGY
North Africa and Middle East	North Africa and Middle East	Iran	IRN
North Africa and Middle East	North Africa and Middle East	Iraq	IRQ
North Africa and Middle East	North Africa and Middle East	Jordan	JOR
North Africa and Middle East	North Africa and Middle East	Kuwait	KWT
North Africa and Middle East	North Africa and Middle East	Lebanon	LBN
North Africa and Middle East	North Africa and Middle East	Libya	LBY
North Africa and Middle East	North Africa and Middle East	Morocco	MAR
North Africa and Middle East	North Africa and Middle East	Occupied Palestinian Territory	PSE
North Africa and Middle East	North Africa and Middle East	Oman	OMN
North Africa and Middle East	North Africa and Middle East	Qatar	QAT

Table A.1. (continued)

GBD superregion	GDB region	Country	ISO3
North Africa and Middle East	North Africa and Middle East	Saudi Arabia	SAU
North Africa and Middle East	North Africa and Middle East	Syria	SYR
North Africa and Middle East	North Africa and Middle East	Tunisia	TUN
North Africa and Middle East	North Africa and Middle East	Turkey	TUR
North Africa and Middle East	North Africa and Middle East	United Arab Emirates	ARE
North Africa and Middle East	North Africa and Middle East	Yemen	YEM
South Asia	South Asia	Bangladesh	BGD
South Asia	South Asia	Bhutan	BTN
South Asia	South Asia	India	IND
South Asia	South Asia	Nepal	NPL
South Asia	South Asia	Pakistan	PAK
Southeast Asia, East Asia, and Oceania	East Asia	China	CHN
Southeast Asia, East Asia, and Oceania	East Asia	Hong Kong Special Administrative Region of China	HKG
Southeast Asia, East Asia, and Oceania	East Asia	North Korea	PRK
Southeast Asia, East Asia, and Oceania	East Asia	Macao Special Administrative Region of China	MAC
Southeast Asia, East Asia, and Oceania	East Asia	Taiwan	TWN
Southeast Asia, East Asia, and Oceania	Oceania	Fiji	FJI

Table A.1. (continued)

GBD superregion	GDB region	Country	ISO3
Southeast Asia, East Asia, and Oceania	Oceania	Kiribati	KIR
Southeast Asia, East Asia, and Oceania	Oceania	Marshall Islands	MHL
Southeast Asia, East Asia, and Oceania	Oceania	Federated States of Micronesia	FSM
Southeast Asia, East Asia, and Oceania	Oceania	Papua New Guinea	PNG
Southeast Asia, East Asia, and Oceania	Oceania	Samoa	WSM
Southeast Asia, East Asia, and Oceania	Oceania	Solomon Islands	SLB
Southeast Asia, East Asia, and Oceania	Oceania	Tonga	TON
Southeast Asia, East Asia, and Oceania	Oceania	Vanuatu	VUT
Southeast Asia, East Asia, and Oceania	Southeast Asia	Cambodia	KHM
Southeast Asia, East Asia, and Oceania	Southeast Asia	Indonesia	IDN
Southeast Asia, East Asia, and Oceania	Southeast Asia	Laos	LAO
Southeast Asia, East Asia, and Oceania	Southeast Asia	Malaysia	MYS
Southeast Asia, East Asia, and Oceania	Southeast Asia	Maldives	MDV
Southeast Asia, East Asia, and Oceania	Southeast Asia	Mauritius	MUS
Southeast Asia, East Asia, and Oceania	Southeast Asia	Burma	MMR
Southeast Asia, East Asia, and Oceania	Southeast Asia	Philippines	PHL
Southeast Asia, East Asia, and Oceania	Southeast Asia	Seychelles	SYC

Table A.1. (continued)

GBD superregion	GDB region	Country	ISO3
Southeast Asia, East Asia, and Oceania	Southeast Asia	Sri Lanka	LKA
Southeast Asia, East Asia, and Oceania	Southeast Asia	Thailand	THA
Southeast Asia, East Asia, and Oceania	Southeast Asia	Timor-Leste	TLS
Southeast Asia, East Asia, and Oceania	Southeast Asia	Vietnam	VNM
Sub-Saharan Africa	Central sub-Saharan Africa	Angola	AGO
Sub-Saharan Africa	Central sub-Saharan Africa	Central African Republic	CAF
Sub-Saharan Africa	Central sub-Saharan Africa	Congo	COG
Sub-Saharan Africa	Central sub-Saharan Africa	Democratic Republic of Congo	COD
Sub-Saharan Africa	Central sub-Saharan Africa	Equatorial Guinea	GNQ
Sub-Saharan Africa	Central sub-Saharan Africa	Gabon	GAB
Sub-Saharan Africa	Eastern sub-Saharan Africa	Burundi	BDI
Sub-Saharan Africa	Eastern sub-Saharan Africa	Comoros	COM
Sub-Saharan Africa	Eastern sub-Saharan Africa	Djibouti	DJI
Sub-Saharan Africa	Eastern sub-Saharan Africa	Eritrea	ERI
Sub-Saharan Africa	Eastern sub-Saharan Africa	Ethiopia	ETH
Sub-Saharan Africa	Eastern sub-Saharan Africa	Kenya	KEN

Table A.1. (continued)

GBD superregion	GDB region	Country	ISO3
Sub-Saharan Africa	Eastern sub-Saharan Africa	Madagascar	MDG
Sub-Saharan Africa	Eastern sub-Saharan Africa	Malawi	MWI
Sub-Saharan Africa	Eastern sub-Saharan Africa	Mozambique	MOZ
Sub-Saharan Africa	Eastern sub-Saharan Africa	Rwanda	RWA
Sub-Saharan Africa	Eastern sub-Saharan Africa	Somalia	SOM
Sub-Saharan Africa	Eastern sub-Saharan Africa	Sudan	SDN
Sub-Saharan Africa	Eastern sub-Saharan Africa	Tanzania	TZA
Sub-Saharan Africa	Eastern sub-Saharan Africa	Uganda	UGA
Sub-Saharan Africa	Eastern sub-Saharan Africa	Zambia	ZMB
Sub-Saharan Africa	Southern sub-Saharan Africa	Botswana	BWA
Sub-Saharan Africa	Southern sub-Saharan Africa	Lesotho	LSO
Sub-Saharan Africa	Southern sub-Saharan Africa	Namibia	NAM
Sub-Saharan Africa	Southern sub-Saharan Africa	South Africa	ZAF
Sub-Saharan Africa	Southern sub-Saharan Africa	Swaziland	SWZ
Sub-Saharan Africa	Southern sub-Saharan Africa	Zimbabwe	ZWE
Sub-Saharan Africa	Western sub-Saharan Africa	Benin	BEN
Sub-Saharan Africa	Western sub-Saharan Africa	Burkina Faso	BFA

Table A.1. (continued)

GBD superregion	GDB region	Country	ISO3
Sub-Saharan Africa	Western sub-Saharan Africa	Cameroon	CMR
Sub-Saharan Africa	Western sub-Saharan Africa	Cape Verde	CPV
Sub-Saharan Africa	Western sub-Saharan Africa	Chad	TCD
Sub-Saharan Africa	Western sub-Saharan Africa	Côte d'Ivoire	CIV
Sub-Saharan Africa	Western sub-Saharan Africa	Gambia	GMB
Sub-Saharan Africa	Western sub-Saharan Africa	Ghana	GHA
Sub-Saharan Africa	Western sub-Saharan Africa	Guinea	GIN
Sub-Saharan Africa	Western sub-Saharan Africa	Guinea-Bissau	GNB
Sub-Saharan Africa	Western sub-Saharan Africa	Liberia	LBR
Sub-Saharan Africa	Western sub-Saharan Africa	Mali	MLI
Sub-Saharan Africa	Western sub-Saharan Africa	Mauritania	MRT
Sub-Saharan Africa	Western sub-Saharan Africa	Niger	NER
Sub-Saharan Africa	Western sub-Saharan Africa	Nigeria	NGA
Sub-Saharan Africa	Western sub-Saharan Africa	SãoTomé and Príncipe	STP
Sub-Saharan Africa	Western sub-Saharan Africa	Senegal	SEN
Sub-Saharan Africa	Western sub-Saharan Africa	Sierra Leone	SLE
Sub-Saharan Africa	Western sub-Saharan Africa	Togo	TGO

References

[1]   Murray CJ, Ezzati M, Flaxman AD, Lim S, Lozano R, Michaud C, et al. GBD 2010: a multi-investigator collaboration for global comparative descriptive epidemiology. The Lancet. 2012;380(9859):2055–2058.

[2]   Murray CJ, Ezzati M, Flaxman AD, Lim S, Lozano R, Michaud C, et al. GBD 2010: design, definitions, and metrics. The Lancet. 2012;380(9859):2063–2066.

[3]   Salomon JA, Vos T, Hogan DR, Gagnon M, Naghavi M, Mokdad A, et al. Common values in assessing health outcomes from disease and injury: disability weights measurement study for the Global Burden of Disease Study 2010. The Lancet. 2012;380(9859):2129–2143.

[4]   Murray CJ, Vos T, Lozano R, Naghavi M, Flaxman AD, Michaud C, et al. Disability-adjusted life years (DALYs) for 291 diseases and injuries in 21 regions, 1990–2010: a systematic analysis for the Global Burden of Disease Study 2010. The Lancet. 2012;380(9859):2197–2223.

[5]   Lozano R, Naghavi M, Foreman K, Lim S, Shibuya K, Aboyans V, et al. Global and regional mortality from 235 causes of death for 20 age groups in 1990 and 2010: a systematic analysis for the Global Burden of Disease Study 2010. The Lancet. 2012;380(9859):2095–2128.

[6]   Vos T, Flaxman A, Naghavi M, Lozano R, Michaud C, Ezzati M, et al. Years lived with disability (YLDs) for 1160 sequelae of 289 diseases and injuries 1990-2010: a systematic analysis for the Global Burden of Disease Study 2010. The Lancet. 2012;380(9859):2163–2196.

[7]   Lim SS, Vos T, Flaxman AD, Danaei G, Shibuya K, Adair-Rohani H, et al. A comparative risk assessment of burden of disease and injury

attributable to 67 risk factors and risk factor clusters in 21 regions, 1990–2010: a systematic analysis for the Global Burden of Disease Study 2010. The Lancet. 2012;380(9859):2224–2260.

[8]   Murray C, Lopez A. Quantifying disability: data, methods and results. Bulletin of the World Health Organization. 1994;72(3):481–494. PMID: 8062403. Available from: http://www.ncbi.nlm.nih.gov/pubmed/8062403.

[9]   Barendregt J, Van Oortmarssen G, Vos T, Murray C. A generic model for the assessment of disease epidemiology: the computational basis of DisMod II. Population Health Metrics. 2003 Apr;1(1):4. PMID: 12773212. Available from: http://www.ncbi.nlm.nih.gov/pubmed/12773212.

[10]   Borenstein M, Hedges L, Higgins J, Rothstein H. Introduction to Meta-Analysis. John Wiley & Sons; 2011.

[11]   DerSimonian R, Laird N. Meta-analysis in clinical trials. Controlled Clinical Trials. 1986;7(3):177–188.

[12]   Stroup DF, Berlin JA, Morton SC, Olkin I, Williamson GD, Rennie D, et al. Meta-analysis of observational studies in epidemiology. JAMA: The Journal of the American Medical Association. 2000;283(15):2008–2012.

[13]   Poewe W. The natural history of Parkinson's disease. Journal of Neurology. 2006 Dec;253 Suppl 7:VII2–6. PMID: 17131223. Available from: http://www.ncbi.nlm.nih.gov/pubmed/17131223.

[14]   Pollock M, Hornabrook R. The prevalence, natural history and dementia of Parkinson's disease. Brain: A Journal of Neurology. 1966 Sep;89(3):429–448. PMID: 5921126. Available from: http://www.ncbi.nlm.nih.gov/pubmed/5921126.

[15]   Larsen J, Dupont E, Tandberg E. Clinical diagnosis of Parkinson's disease. Proposal of diagnostic subgroups classified at different levels of confidence. Acta Neurologica Scandinavica. 1994 Apr;89(4):242–251. PMID: 8042440. Available from: http://www.ncbi.nlm.nih.gov/pubmed/8042440.

[16] Mutch WJ, Dingwall-Fordyce I, Downie AW, Paterson JG, Roy SK. Parkinson's disease in a Scottish city. British Medical Journal (Clinical research ed). 1986;292(6519):534.

[17] Benito-León J, Bermejo-Pareja F, Morales-Gonzalez J, Porta-Etessam J, Trincado R, Vega S, et al. Incidence of Parkinson disease and parkinsonism in three elderly populations of central Spain. Neurology. 2004;62(5):734–741.

[18] Kuroda K, Tatara K, Shinsho H, Okamoto E, Cho R, Nishigaki C, et al. [A study of attitudes toward illness and its effect on mortality in patients with Parkinson's disease]. [Nihon koshu eisei zasshi] Japanese Journal of Public Health. 1990;37(5):333–339.

[19] Foreman K, Lozano R, Lopez A, Murray C. Modeling causes of death: an integrated approach using CODEm. Population Health Metrics. 2012;10:1. PMID: 22226226. Available from: http://www.ncbi.nlm.nih.gov/pubmed/22226226.

[20] Pearson K. Report on certain enteric fever inoculation statistics. British Medical Journal. 1904 Nov;2(2288):1243–1246. PMID: 20761760 PMCID: 2355479.

[21] Larsen P, von Ins M. The rate of growth in scientific publication and the decline in coverage provided by Science Citation Index. Scientometrics. 2010 Sep;84(3):575–603. PMID: 20700371 PMCID: 2909426.

[22] {US National Library of Medicine National Institutes of Health}. PubMed; 2012. http://www.ncbi.nlm.nih.gov/pubmed. Available from: http://www.ncbi.nlm.nih.gov/pubmed.

[23] The Cochrane Collaboration; 2012. http://www.cochrane.org/. Available from: http://www.cochrane.org/.

[24] Green S. Systematic reviews and meta-analysis. Singapore Medical Journal. 2005 Jun;46(6):270–273; quiz 274. PMID: 15902354. Available from: http://www.ncbi.nlm.nih.gov/pubmed/15902354.

[25] Moher D, Liberati A, Tetzlaff J, Altman D, Group TP. Preferred Reporting Items for Systematic Reviews and Meta-Analyses: The PRISMA Statement. PLoS Medicine. 2009 Jul;6(7):e1000097. Available from: http://dx.doi.org/10.1371/journal.pmed.1000097.

[26] for Applied Systems Analysis II, Klementiev A. On the Estimation
      of Morbidity. Laxenburg Austria: International Institute for Applied
      Systems Analysis; 1977.

[27] Murray C, Lopez A. The Global Burden of Disease: A Comprehensive
      Assessment of Mortality and Disability from Diseases, Injuries, and Risk
      Factors in 1990 and Projected to 2020. Cambridge MA: Published by
      the Harvard School of Public Health on behalf of the World Health
      Organization and the World Bank; Distributed by Harvard University
      Press; 1996.

[28] Lozano R.   Burden of disease assessment and health system reform:
      results of a study in Mexico. Journal of International Development.
      1995;7(3):555.

[29] {Republica de Colombia Ministerio de Salud}. La carga de la enfermedad
      en Colombia. 7th ed. Santafe de Bogota: Editorial Carrera; 1994.

[30] Concha Barrientos M, Aguilera Sanhueza X, Salas Vergara J. La Carga
      de Enfermedad en Chile.   Ministerio de Salud Republica de Chile;
      1996.   Available from: http://epi.minsal.cl/epi/html/sdesalud/carga/
      Inffin-carga-enf.pdf.

[31] Vos T, Timaeus I, Gareeboo J, Roussety F, Huttly S, Murray C. Mauri-
      tius Health Sector Reform, National Burden of Disease Study. Mauritius
      Ministry of Health and Ministry of Economic Planning; 1996. Available
      from: http://espace.library.uq.edu.au/view/UQ:155551.

[32] Bundhamchareon K, Teerawattananon Y, Vos T, Begg S. Burden of
      disease and injuries in Thailand. Nonthaburi, Thailand: Ministry of
      Public Health. Ministry of Public Health; 2002.

[33] Yusoff A, Mustafa A, Kaur G, Omar M, Vos T, Rao V, et al. Malaysian
      Burden of Disease and Injury Study. In: Forum 9; 2005. p. 1–24.

[34] Chapman G, Hansen KS, Jelsma J, Ndhlovu C, Piotti B, Byskov J,
      et al. The burden of disease in Zimbabwe in 1997 as measured by
      disability-adjusted life years lost. Tropical Medicine & International
      Health. 2006;11(5):660–671.

[35] Begg SJ, Vos T, Barker B, Stanley L, Lopez AD. Burden of disease and injury in Australia in the new millennium: measuring health loss from diseases, injuries and risk factors. Medical Journal of Australia. 2008;188(1):36.

[36] Tanner M. From EM to data augmentation: The emergence of MCMC Bayesian computation in the 1980s. Statistical Science. 2010;25(4):506–506 516.

[37] Gelman A, Carlin J, Stern H, Rubin D. Bayesian Data Analysis, Second Edition. 2nd ed. Chapman and Hall/CRC; 2003.

[38] Carlin BP, Louis TA. Bayes and Empirical Bayes Methods for Data Analysis. CRC Press; 2010.

[39] Jaynes ET. Probability Theory: The Logic of Science. Cambridge University Press; 2003.

[40] Mayo DG. Error and the Growth of Experimental Knowledge. University of Chicago Press; 1996.

[41] Robert C. The Bayesian Choice: From Decision-Theoretic Foundations to Computational Implementation. Springer; 2007.

[42] Collaboration APCS. The effects of diabetes on the risks of major cardiovascular diseases and death in the Asia-Pacific region. Diabetes care. 2003;26(2):360–366.

[43] Rothstein HR, Sutton AJ, Borenstein M. Publication Bias in Meta-Analysis: Prevention, Assessment and Adjustments. John Wiley & Sons; 2005.

[44] Rabe-Hesketh W, Skrondal A. Multilevel and Longitudinal Modeling Using Stata. Stata Press; 2008.

[45] Girosi F, King G. Demographic Forecasting. Princeton: Princeton University Press; 2008.

[46] Hogan MC, Foreman KJ, Naghavi M, Ahn SY, Wang M, Makela SM, et al. Maternal mortality for 181 countries, 19802008: a systematic analysis of progress towards Millennium Development Goal 5. The Lancet.

2010;375(9726):1609–1623. Available from: http://www.sciencedirect.com/science/article/pii/S0140673610605181.

[47] Rajaratnam J, Marcus J, Flaxman A, Wang H, Levin-Rector A, Dwyer L, et al. Neonatal, postneonatal, childhood, and under-5 mortality for 187 countries, 19702010: a systematic analysis of progress towards Millennium Development Goal 4. The Lancet. 2010;375(9730):1988–2008. Available from: http://www.sciencedirect.com/science/article/pii/S0140673610607039.

[48] Hastie T, Tibshirani R, Friedman JH. The Elements of Statistical Learning: Data Mining, Inference, and Prediction. Springer; 2009.

[49] Wahba G. Spline Models for Observational Data. Philadelphia Pa.: Society for Industrial and Applied Mathematics; 1990.

[50] Danaei G. National, regional, and global trends in systolic blood pressure since 1980: Systematic analysis of health examination surveys and epidemiological studies with 786 country-years and 5.4 million participants. The Lancet. 2011;377(9765):568–568–577.

[51] Raftery A, Madigan D, Hoeting J. Bayesian model averaging for linear regression models. Journal of the American Statistical Association. 1997;92(437):179–191. Available from: http://www.tandfonline.com/doi/abs/10.1080/01621459.1997.10473615.

[52] Friedman J. Multivariate Adaptive Regression Splines. The Annals of Statistics. 1991 Mar;19(1). Available from: http://projecteuclid.org/euclid.aos/1176347963.

[53] Dierckx P. Curve and Surface Fitting with Splines. Oxford University Press; 1995.

[54] Rasmussen C, Williams C. Gaussian Processes for Machine Learning. MIT Press; 2006.

[55] Diggle P, Ribeiro P. Model-Based Geostatistics. Springer; 2010.

[56] Neal RM. 5. In: MCMC using Hamiltonian dynamics. Taylor & Francis US; 2011.

[57] Hoffman MD, Gelman A. The no-U-turn sampler: adaptively setting path lengths in Hamiltonian Monte Carlo. arXiv preprint arXiv:11114246. 2011.

[58] Goodman J, Weare J. Ensemble Samplers with Affine Invariance. Communications in Applied Mathematics and Computational Science. 2010;5(1):65–80.

[59] Papp D, Alizadeh F. Shape constrained estimation using nonnegative splines. Journal of Computational and Graphical Statistics. 2012.

[60] Amemiya T. Regression analysis when the dependent variable is truncated normal. Econometrica. 1973 Nov;41(6). Available from: http://www.jstor.org/stable/1914031.

[61] Manski C, Tamer E. Inference on regressions with interval data on a regressor or outcome. Econometrica. 2002;70(2):519546.

[62] Cook J, McDonald J. Partially adaptive estimation of interval censored regression models. Computational Economics. 2012;40(1):1–13. Available from: http://www.springerlink.com/content/244658nl438rk904/abstract/.

[63] Greenwood M. Proceedings of a meeting of the Royal Statistical Society held on July 16th, 1946. Journal of the Royal Statistical Society. 1946;109(4):pp. 325–378. Available from: http://www.jstor.org/stable/2981330.

[64] Forrester J. Industrial dynamics. Cambridge Mass.: MIT Press; 1961. [65]

Forrester J. Urban Dynamics. Cambridge Mass.: MIT Press; 1969.

[66] Forrester J. World Dynamics. Wright-Allen Press; 1973.

[67] Meadows D. Thinking in Systems: A Primer. White River Junction Vt.: Chelsea Green Pub.; 2008.

[68] Hethcote H. Qualitative analyses of communicable disease models. Mathematical Biosciences. 1976;28(3-4):335–335–356.

[69] Anderson R, May R. Infectious Diseases of Humans: Dynamics and Control. Oxford University Press; 1992.

[70] Diekmann O, Heesterbeek J. Mathematical Epidemiology of Infectious Diseases: Model Building, Analysis, and Interpretation. John Wiley and Sons; 2000.

[71] Keeling MJ, Rohani P. Modeling Infectious Diseases in Humans and Animals. Princeton University Press; 2008.

[72] Vynnycky E, White R. An Introduction to Infectious Disease Modelling. Oxford University Press; 2010.

[73] Sheiner L, Rosenberg B, Melmon K. Modelling of individual pharmacokinetics for computer-aided drug dosage. Computers and Biomedical Research. 1972 Oct;5(5):441–459. Available from: http://www.sciencedirect.com/science/article/pii/0010480972900511.

[74] Jacquez JA. Compartmental Analysis in Biology and Medicine. University of Michigan Press; 1985.

[75] Yuh L, A S, Davidian M, Harrison F, Hester A, Kowalski K, et al. Population pharmacokinetic/pharmacodynamic methodology and applications: a bibliography. Biometrics. 1994 Jun;50(2). Available from: http://www.jstor.org/stable/2533402.

[76] Barrett P, Bell B, Cobelli C, Golde H, Schumitzky A, Vicini P, et al. SAAM II: Simulation, analysis, and modeling software for tracer and pharmacokinetic studies. Metabolism. 1998 Apr;47(4):484–492. Available from: http://www.sciencedirect.com/science/article/pii/S0026049598900646.

[77] Jacquez JA. Modeling with Compartments. BioMedware; 1999.

[78] Atkinson AJ, Lalonde R. Introduction of quantitative methods in pharmacology and clinical pharmacology: a historical overview. Clinical Pharmacology and Therapeutics. 2007 Jul;82(1):3–6. PMID: 17571065. Available from: http://www.ncbi.nlm.nih.gov/pubmed/17571065.

[79] Harte J. Consider a Spherical Cow. University Science Books; 1988.

[80] Richardson G. Feedback Thought in Social Science and Systems Theory. Philadelphia: University of Pennsylvania Press; 1991.

[81] Wang H, Dwyer-Lindgren L, Lofgren K, Rajaratnam J, Marcus J, Levin-Rector A, et al. Age-specific and sex-specific mortality in 187 countries, 1970–2010: a systematic analysis for the Global Burden of Disease Study 2010. The Lancet. 2012;380:2071–2094.

[82] Williams J. From Sails to Satellites: The Origin and Development of Navigational Science. Oxford University Press, USA; 1993.

[83] Legendre A. Nouvelles Mthodes Pour La Dtermination Des Orbites Des Comtes. Ulan Press; 2011.

[84] Eckhardt R. Stan Ulam, John Von Neumann, and the Monte Carlo Method. Los Alamos Science. 1987;15(Special Issue):131–143.

[85] Geman S, Geman D. Stochastic relaxation, Gibbs distributions, and the Bayesian restoration of images. Pattern Analysis and Machine Intelligence, IEEE Transactions on. 1984;PAMI-6(6):721–741.

[86] Gelfand AE, Smith AFM. Sampling-based approaches to calculating marginal densities. Journal of the American Statistical Association. 1990;85(410):pp. 398–409. Available from: http://www.jstor.org/stable/2289776.

[87] Dyer M, Frieze A, Kannan R. A random polynomial-time algorithm for approximating the volume of convex bodies. Journal of the ACM. 1991 Jan;38(1):117. Available from: http://doi.acm.org/10.1145/102782.102783.

[88] Lováz L, Vempala S. Hit-and-run from a corner. Proceedings of the Thiry-sixth Annual ACM Symposium on Theory of Computing. 2004;p. 310–314.

[89] Metropolis N, Rosenbluth A, Rosenbluth M, Teller A, Teller E. Equation of state calculations by fast computing machines. The Journal of Chemical Physics. 1953;21(6):1087–1092.

[90] Hastings WK. Monte Carlo sampling methods using Markov chains and their applications. Biometrika. 1970 Apr;57(1):97–109. Available from: http://biomet.oxfordjournals.org/content/57/1/97.

[91] Chib S, Greenberg E. Understanding the Metropolis-Hastings algorithm. The American Statistician. 1995;49(4):327–335.

[92] Haario H. An adaptive Metropolis algorithm. Bernoulli. 2001;7(2):223.

[93] Powell M. An efficient method for finding the minimum of a function of several variables without calculating derivatives. The Computer Journal. 1964 Jan;7(2):155–162.

[94] Matsumoto M, Nishimura T. Mersenne twister: a 623-dimensionally equidistributed uniform pseudo-random number generator. ACM Transactions on Modeling and Computer Simulation. 1998 Jan;8(1):330. Available from: http://doi.acm.org/10.1145/272991.272995.

[95] Patil A, Huard D, Fonnesbeck CJ. PyMC: Bayesian Stochastic modelling in Python. Journal of Statistical Software. 2010;35(4):1–1–81.

[96] Gelman A, Roberts G, Gilks W. Efficient Metropolis jumping rules. In: Bayesian Statistics V. Oxford: Oxford University Press; 1996. p. 599–608.

[97] Gilks W, Roberts G, George E. Adaptive direction sampling. The Statistician. 1994;p. 179189. Available from: http://www.jstor.org/stable/10.2307/2348942.

[98] Gilks WR, Roberts GO, Sahu SK. Adaptive Markov chain Monte Carlo through regeneration. Journal of the American Statistical Association. 1998;93(443):1045–1054. Available from: http://www.tandfonline.com/doi/abs/10.1080/01621459.1998.10473766.

[99] Sahu S, Zhigljavsky A. Self regenerative Markov chain Monte Carlo with adaptation. Preprint; 1999. Available from: http://www.statslab.cam.ac.uk/~mcmc.

[100] Bubley R, Dyer M. Path coupling: a technique for proving rapid mixing in Markov chains. In: , 38th Annual Symposium on Foundations of Computer Science, 1997. Proceedings; 1997. p. 223 –231.

[101] Dyer M, Greenhill C. On Markov chains for independent sets. Journal of Algorithms. 2000 Apr;35(1):17–49. Available from: http://www.sciencedirect.com/science/article/pii/S0196677499910714.

[102] Geyer C. Introduction to Markov-chain monte carlo. In: Handbook of Markov Chain Monte Carlo. CRC Press; 2010. p. 30.

[103] Bhatnagar N, Bogdanov A, Mossel E. The Computational Complexity of Estimating MCMC Convergence Time. In: Goldberg L, Jansen K, Ravi R, Rolim J, editors. Approximation, Randomization, and Combinatorial Optimization. Algorithms and Techniques. vol. 6845 of Lecture Notes in Computer Science. Springer Berlin / Heidelberg; 2011. p. 424–435. Available from: http://www.springerlink.com/content/45tqr1467x706852/abstract/.

[104] Gilks WR, Richardson S, Spiegelhalter DJ. Markov Chain Monte Carlo in Practice. CRC Press; 1996.

[105] Wakefield J, Bennett J. The Bayesian Modeling of Covariates for Population Pharmacokinetic Models. Journal of the American Statistical Association. 1996;91(435). Available from: http://www.jstor.org/stable/2291710.

[106] Mengersen K, Robert C, Guihenneuc-Jouyaux C. MCMC Convergence Diagnostics: A Review. In: Bayesian Statistics 6. Oxford University Press; 1999. p. 415–440.

[107] Lovsz L. Hit-and-run mixes fast. Mathematical Programming. 1999;86(3):443–461. Available from: http://www.springerlink.com/content/u36kvcmgrvjta7ql/abstract/.

[108] Kannan R, Lovsz L, Simonovits M. Random walks and O*(n5) volume algorithm for convex bodies. Random Strucutres & Algorithms. 1997 Jan;11:1–50.

[109] Gelman A. Inference from iterative simulation using multiple sequences. Statistical Science. 1992 Nov;7(4):457–472. Available from: http://projecteuclid.org/euclid.ss/1177011136.

[110] Frieze A, Kannan R, Polson N. Sampling from log-concave distributions. The Annals of Applied Probability. 1994;4(3). Available from: http://www.jstor.org/stable/2245065.

[111] Jennison C. Discussion on the Gibbs sampler and the other Markov chain Monte Carlo methods. Journal of the Royal Statistical Society: Series B. 1993;55(1):54–56.

[112] Brooks S, Gelman A. General methods for monitoring convergence of iterative simulations. Journal of Computational and Graphical Statistics. 1998 Dec;7(4). Available from: http://www.jstor.org/stable/1390675.

[113] Brooks S, Roberts G. Convergence assessment techniques for Markov chain Monte Carlo. Statistics and Computing. 1998;8(4):319–335. Available from: http://www.springerlink.com/content/p74l73t52672h40g/abstract/.

[114] Tseng P. Convergence of a block coordinate descent method for non-differentiable minimization. Journal of Optimization Theory and Applications. 2001;109(3):475–494. Available from: http://www.springerlink.com/content/q327675221126243/abstract/.

[115] Yedidia J, Freeman W, Weiss Y. Generalized Belief Propagation. In: IN NIPS 13. MIT Press; 2000. p. 689–695.

[116] Braunstein A, Mézard M, Zecchina R. Survey propagation: an algorithm for satisfiability. Random Structures & Algorithms. 2005;27(2):201–226.

[117] Wainwright MJ, Jordan MI. Graphical models, exponential families, and variational inference. Foundations and Trends® in Machine Learning. 2008;1(1-2):1–305.

[118] Bell B, Flaxman A. A statistical model and estimation of disease rates as functions of age and time. SIAM Journal on Scientific Computing;35(2).

[119] Association AP. Diagnostic and Statistical Manual of Mental Disorders, Fourth Edition: DSM-IV-TR. American Psychiatric Pub; 2000.

[120] Wagner F, Anthony J. From first drug use to drug dependence; developmental periods of risk for dependence upon marijuana, cocaine, and alcohol. Neuropsychopharmacology: Official Publication of the American College of Neuropsychopharmacology. 2002 Apr;26(4):479–488. PMID: 11927172. Available from: http://www.ncbi.nlm.nih.gov/pubmed/11927172.

[121] Degenhardt L, Bucello C, Calabria B, Nelson P, Roberts A, Hall W, et al. What data are available on the extent of illicit drug use and dependence globally? Results of four systematic reviews. Drug and Alcohol Dependence. 2011 Sep;117(2-3):85–101. PMID: 21377813. Available from: http://www.ncbi.nlm.nih.gov/pubmed/21377813.

[122] Spiegelhalter DJ, Best NG, Carlin BP, van der Linde A. Bayesian measures of model complexity and fit. Journal of the Royal Statistical Society: Series B (Statistical Methodology). 2002;64(4):583–639. Available from: http://dx.doi.org/10.1111/1467-9868.00353.

[123] Dickerson L, Mazyck P, Hunter M. Premenstrual syndrome. American Family Physician. 2003 Apr;67(8):1743–1752. PMID: 12725453. Available from: http://www.ncbi.nlm.nih.gov/pubmed/12725453.

[124] Singh B, Berman B, Simpson R, Annechild A. Incidence of premenstrual syndrome and remedy usage: a national probability sample study. Alternative Therapies in Health and Medicine. 1998 May;4(3):75–79. PMID: 9581324. Available from: http://www.ncbi.nlm.nih.gov/pubmed/9581324.

[125] Goodale I, Domar A, Benson H. Alleviation of premenstrual syndrome symptoms with the relaxation response. Obstetrics and Gynecology. 1990 Apr;75(4):649–655. PMID: 2179779. Available from: http://www.ncbi.nlm.nih.gov/pubmed/2179779.

[126] Raraty M, Connor S, Criddle D, Sutton R, Neoptolemos J. Acute pancreatitis and organ failure: pathophysiology, natural history, and management strategies. Current Gastroenterology Reports. 2004;6(2):99–103. Available from: http://www.springerlink.com/content/2p5825613213409n/abstract/.

[127] Banks P. Epidemiology, natural history, and predictors of disease outcome in acute and chronic pancreatitis. Gastrointestinal Endoscopy. 2002 Dec;56(6 Suppl):S226–230. PMID: 12447272. Available from: http://www.ncbi.nlm.nih.gov/pubmed/12447272.

[128] Sekimoto M, Takada T, Kawarada Y, Hirata K, Mayumi T, Yoshida M, et al. JPN Guidelines for the management of acute pancreatitis: epidemiology, etiology, natural history, and outcome predictors in acute pancreatitis. Journal of Hepato-Biliary-Pancreatic Surgery. 2006 Feb;13(1):10–24. PMID: 16463207 PMCID: PMC2779368. Available from: http://www.ncbi.nlm.nih.gov/pmc/articles/PMC2779368/.

[129] Rich M. Epidemiology of atrial fibrillation. Journal of Interventional Cardiac Electrophysiology: An International Journal of Arrhythmias

and Pacing. 2009 Jun;25(1):3–8. PMID: 19160031. Available from: http://www.ncbi.nlm.nih.gov/pubmed/19160031.

[130] Rho R, Page R. Asymptomatic atrial fibrillation. Progress in Cardiovascular Diseases. 2005 Oct;48(2):79–87. PMID: 16253649. Available from: http://www.ncbi.nlm.nih.gov/pubmed/16253649.

[131] Fuster V, Rydn L, Cannom D, Crijns H, Curtis A, Ellenbogen K, et al. ACC/AHA/ESC 2006 Guidelines for the Management of Patients With Atrial FibrillationExecutive Summary. Journal of the American College of Cardiology. 2006 Aug;48(4):854–906. Available from: http://content.onlinejacc.org/article.aspx?volume=48&issueno=4&page=854.

[132] Radford D, Izukawa T. Atrial fibrillation in children. Pediatrics. 1977 Feb;59(2):250–256. PMID: 834508. Available from: http://www.ncbi.nlm.nih.gov/pubmed/834508.

[133] Hoofnagle JH. Hepatitis C: the clinical spectrum of disease. Hepatology. 1997 Sep;26(3 Suppl 1):15S–20S. PMID: 9305658. Available from: http://www.ncbi.nlm.nih.gov/pubmed/9305658.

[134] Ghany M, Strader D, Thomas D, Seeff L. Diagnosis, management, and treatment of hepatitis C: an update. Hepatology. 2009 Apr;49(4):1335–1374. PMID: 19330875. Available from: http://www.ncbi.nlm.nih.gov/pubmed/19330875.

[135] Ghany M, Nelson D, Strader D, Thomas D, Seeff L. An update on treatment of genotype 1 chronic hepatitis C virus infection: 2011 practice guideline by the American Association for the Study of Liver Diseases. Hepatology. 2011 Oct;54(4):1433–1444. PMID: 21898493. Available from: http://www.ncbi.nlm.nih.gov/pubmed/21898493.

[136] Frank C, Mohamed M, Strickland G, Lavanchy D, Arthur R, Magder L, et al. The role of parenteral antischistosomal therapy in the spread of hepatitis C virus in Egypt. The Lancet. 2000 Mar;355(9207):887–891. PMID: 10752705. Available from: http://www.ncbi.nlm.nih.gov/pubmed/10752705.

[137] Mezban Z, Wakil A. Hepatitis C in Egypt. American Journal of Gastroenterology. 2006;.

[138] Strickland G. Liver disease in Egypt: hepatitis C superseded schistosomiasis as a result of iatrogenic and biological factors. Hepatology. 2006 May;43(5):915–922. PMID: 16628669. Available from: http://www.ncbi.nlm.nih.gov/pubmed/16628669.

[139] Garcia-Tsao G, Lim J, Lim J. Management and treatment of patients with cirrhosis and portal hypertension: recommendations from the Department of Veterans Affairs Hepatitis C Resource Center Program and the National Hepatitis C Program. The American Journal of Gastroenterology. 2009 Jul;104(7):1802–1829. PMID: 19455106. Available from: http://www.ncbi.nlm.nih.gov/pubmed/19455106.

[140] D'Amico G, Garcia-Tsao G, Pagliaro L. Natural history and prognostic indicators of survival in cirrhosis: a systematic review of 118 studies. Journal of Hepatology. 2006 Jan;44(1):217–231. PMID: 16298014. Available from: http://www.ncbi.nlm.nih.gov/pubmed/16298014.

[141] Schuppan D, Afdhal N. Liver cirrhosis. The Lancet. 2008 Mar;371(9615):838–851. PMID: 18328931. Available from: http://www.ncbi.nlm.nih.gov/pubmed/18328931.

[142] He FJ, Nowson CA, Lucas M, MacGregor GA. Increased consumption of fruit and vegetables is related to a reduced risk of coronary heart disease: meta-analysis of cohort studies. Journal of Human Hypertension. 2007 Sep;21(9):717–728. PMID: 17443205. Available from: http://www.ncbi.nlm.nih.gov/pubmed/17443205.

[143] Boeing H, Dietrich T, Hoffmann K, Pischon T, Ferrari P, Lahmann P, et al. Intake of fruits and vegetables and risk of cancer of the upper aerodigestive tract: the prospective EPIC-study. Cancer Causes & Control: CCC. 2006 Sep;17(7):957–969. PMID: 16841263. Available from: http://www.ncbi.nlm.nih.gov/pubmed/16841263.

[144] Banerjee S, Gelfand AE, Carlin BP. Hierarchical modeling and analysis for spatial data. CRC Press; 2003.

[145] K/DOQI clinical practice guidelines for chronic kidney disease: evaluation, classification, and stratification. American Journal of Kidney Diseases: The Official Journal of the National Kidney Foundation. 2002 Feb;39(2 Suppl 1):S1–266. PMID: 11904577. Available from: http://www.ncbi.nlm.nih.gov/pubmed/11904577.

[146] DiPiro J, Talbert RL, Yee GC, Matzke GR, Wells BG, Posey L. Pharmacotherapy: A Pathophysiologic Approach. 7th ed. China: McGraw-Hill Companies; 2008.

[147] Felson D. Epidemiology of hip and knee osteoarthritis. Epidemiologic Reviews. 1988;10:1–28. PMID: 3066625. Available from: http://www.ncbi.nlm.nih.gov/pubmed/3066625.

[148] Felson D, Zhang Y, Hannan M, Naimark A, Weissman B, Aliabadi P, et al. The incidence and natural history of knee osteoarthritis in the elderly. The Framingham Osteoarthritis Study. Arthritis and Rheumatism. 1995 Oct;38(10):1500–1505. PMID: 7575700. Available from: http://www.ncbi.nlm.nih.gov/pubmed/7575700.

[149] Kloos A, Robb A. Bipolar disorder in children and adolescents. Pediatric Annals. 2011 Oct;40(10):481–487. PMID: 21973039. Available from: http://www.ncbi.nlm.nih.gov/pubmed/21973039.

[150] Angst J, Sellaro R. Historical perspectives and natural history of bipolar disorder. Biological Psychiatry. 2000 Sep;48(6):445–457. PMID: 11018218. Available from: http://www.ncbi.nlm.nih.gov/pubmed/11018218.

[151] Hasin DS, Stinson FS, Ogburn E, Grant BF. Prevalence, correlates, disability, and comorbidity of DSM-IV alcohol abuse and dependence in the United States: results from the National Epidemiologic Survey on Alcohol and Related Conditions. Archives of General Psychiatry. 2007 Jul;64(7):830–842. PMID: 17606817. Available from: http://www.ncbi.nlm.nih.gov/pubmed/17606817.

Contributors

Amanda Baxter, MPH
Queensland Centre for Mental Health Research

Jed Blore, PhD
University of Queensland School of Population Health

David Chou, BA
Institute for Health Metrics and Evaluation

Sumeet Chugh, MD
Cedars-Sinai Medical Center

Marita Cross, PhD
University of Sydney

Louisa Degenhardt, PhD
National Drug and Alcohol Research Centre,
University of New South Wales

Alizé Ferrari, PhD
Queensland Centre for Mental Health Research

Abraham D. Flaxman, PhD
Institute for Health Metrics and Evaluation

Mohammad H. Forouzanfar, MD, PhD
Institute for Health Metrics and Evaluation

Justina Groeger, MD, MPH
College of Medicine,
SUNY Downstate Medical Center

Khayriyyah Mohd Hanafiah, MPH
Bloomberg School of Public Health,
Johns Hopkins University

Damian Hoy, PhD
Monash University, Melbourne

Yong Yi Lee, MHEcon
University of Queensland School of Population Health

Stephen S. Lim, PhD
Institute for Health Metrics and Evaluation

Lyn March, PhD
Institute of Bone and Joint Research,
University of Sydney

Ali Mokdad, PhD
Institute for Health Metrics and Evaluation

Christopher J.L. Murray, MD, DPhil
Institute for Health Metrics and Evaluation

Mohsen Naghavi, MD, PhD
Institute for Health Metrics and Evaluation

Hannah M. Peterson, BS
Institute for Health Metrics and Evaluation

Juergen Rehm, PhD
Centre for Addiction and Mental Health, Toronto

Giuseppi Remuzzi, MD
Mario Negri Institute for Pharmacological Research,
Bergamo, Italy

Theo Vos, PhD
Institute for Health Metrics and Evaluation;
University of Queensland School of Population Health

Harvey Whiteford, PhD
Queensland Centre for Mental Health Research

Steven T. Wiersma, MD, MPH
Centers for Disease Control and Prevention

Sarah K. Wulf, MPH
Institute for Health Metrics and Evaluation

About the editors

ABRAHAM FLAXMAN, PhD, is an Assistant Professor of Global Health at the Institute for Health Metrics and Evaluation (IHME) at the University of Washington. He is the primary architect of the software tool DisMod-MR, which IHME uses to estimate the Global Burden of Disease. He and other researchers use the tool to fill in gaps in incomplete data on stroke, malaria, depression, and other diseases from government records and surveys and to correct for inconsistencies.

Prior to being named assistant professor, Dr. Flaxman was a Post-Graduate Fellow at IHME. He previously was a post-doctoral fellow at Microsoft Research.

Originally from Evanston, Illinois, Dr. Flaxman earned his BS in Mathematics from the Massachusetts Institute of Technology. He earned his PhD in Algorithms, Combinatorics, and Optimization from Carnegie Mellon University in 2006.

THEO VOS, MD, MSc, PhD, is a Professor of Global Health at IHME. He is a key member of the Global Burden of Disease (GBD) research team. In this role, he works to improve the GBD methods, update sources of data, and develop partnerships with countries to produce GBD estimates that are most relevant to policy decision-making. He is also focused on linking the epidemiological estimates from GBD to information on health expenditure and cost-effectiveness.

Prior to joining IHME, Dr. Vos was Director of the Centre for Burden of Disease and Cost-Effectiveness at the School of Population Health of the University of Queensland. While there, he led burden of disease studies in Australia and contributed to studies in Malaysia, South Africa, Singapore, Thailand, Vietnam, and Zimbabwe.

Dr. Vos received his PhD in epidemiology and health economics from Erasmus University and his medical degree from State University Groningen, both in the Netherlands. He also studied at the London School of Hygiene and Tropical Medicine, where he obtained an MSc in Public Health in Developing Countries.

CHRISTOPHER J.L. MURRAY, MD, DPhil, is a Professor of Global Health at the University of Washington and Institute Director of IHME whose career has focused on improving health for everyone worldwide by improving health evidence. A physician and health economist, his work has led to the development of a range of new methods and empirical studies to strengthen health measurement, analyze the performance of public health and medical care systems, and assess the cost-effectiveness of health technologies.

Dr. Murray is a founder of the Global Burden of Disease approach, a systematic effort to quantify the comparative magnitude of health loss due to diseases, injuries, and risk factors by age, sex, and geography over time. He led the consortium of researchers that produced the Global Burden of Diseases, Injuries, and Risk Factors Study 2010 (GBD 2010) and continues to direct the GBD enterprise, which now produces annual updates and involves over 1,000 researchers in more than 100 countries.

He holds BA and BS degrees from Harvard University, a DPhil in International Health Economics from Oxford University, and an MD from Harvard Medical School.

Index

A

B

"Ball Walk" algorithm, 94-95

basis functions, piecewise linear spline model, 35–37

Bayesian analysis

data likelihood function, 11–12

empirical priors, pancreatitis case study, 125–128

evolution of, 92–93

hierarchical similarity priors, 48–49

historical background on, 3–4

Metropolis-Hastings step method, 96–97

nonfatal epidemiological data, xx–xxi

Parkinson's disease case study, xxiv–xxx

penalized spline models, 38

smoking prevalence meta-analysis, 4–8, xxiii–xxiv

strength between regions, 102–103

Bayesian information criteria (BIC), spline model of cocaine prevalence, 113–116

beta-binomial model, 30–31

properties of, 18–19

biased estimates, in binomial model, 16–17

binomial model, 13–17, 30–31

bipolar disorder data

cross-walk fixed effects, covariate modeling, 69–71

expert priors, compartmental models, 165–169

C

cause-specific mortality rates (CSMRs)

alcohol dependence studies, 171–174

lower-bound data model, 25–27

Parkinson's disease metaregression, xxvii

transformed normal models and, 25

cirrhosis, out-of-sample predictions, 145–148

cocaine dependence studies, spline models, knot selection, 109–116

Cochrane Collaboration, xxxii–xxxiii

compartmental models

cause-specific mortality rates, alcohol dependency, 171–174

disease in population, two-compartment models, 79–85

end-stage renal disease, 155–159

expert priors, 48, 165–169

future challenges, 88

incidence and prevalence estimates, age group heterogeneity, 131–133

lower-bound data model, 25–27

population dynamics example, 78–79

spline models, knee osteoarthritis, 161–163

compressed estimates, geographical variation, hepatitis C prevalence models, 137–140

convergence, Markov Chain Monte Carlo algorithm, 99–100

coordinate descent, Markov Chain Monte Carlo values, 101

count models, fruit consumption and disease risk, 149–153

covariate modeling, 12, 65–75

consistency and, 74–75

cross-walk fixed effects, bias and, 67–70

evolution of, 65–66

predictive fixed effects, out-of-sample estimation, 71

spatial variation random effects, 72–74

variance analysis, 71–72

cross-validation

heterogeneous age group model comparison, 61–63

model comparisons, 29–31

spine models, 41

cross-walk fixed effects

anxiety disorders prevalence, 141–143

covariate modeling bias and, 67–70

cubic regression spline, age-specific mortality, 37

D

data quality, Parkinson's disease metaregression, xxvii–xxix

design matrix, random effects for spatial variation, 73–74